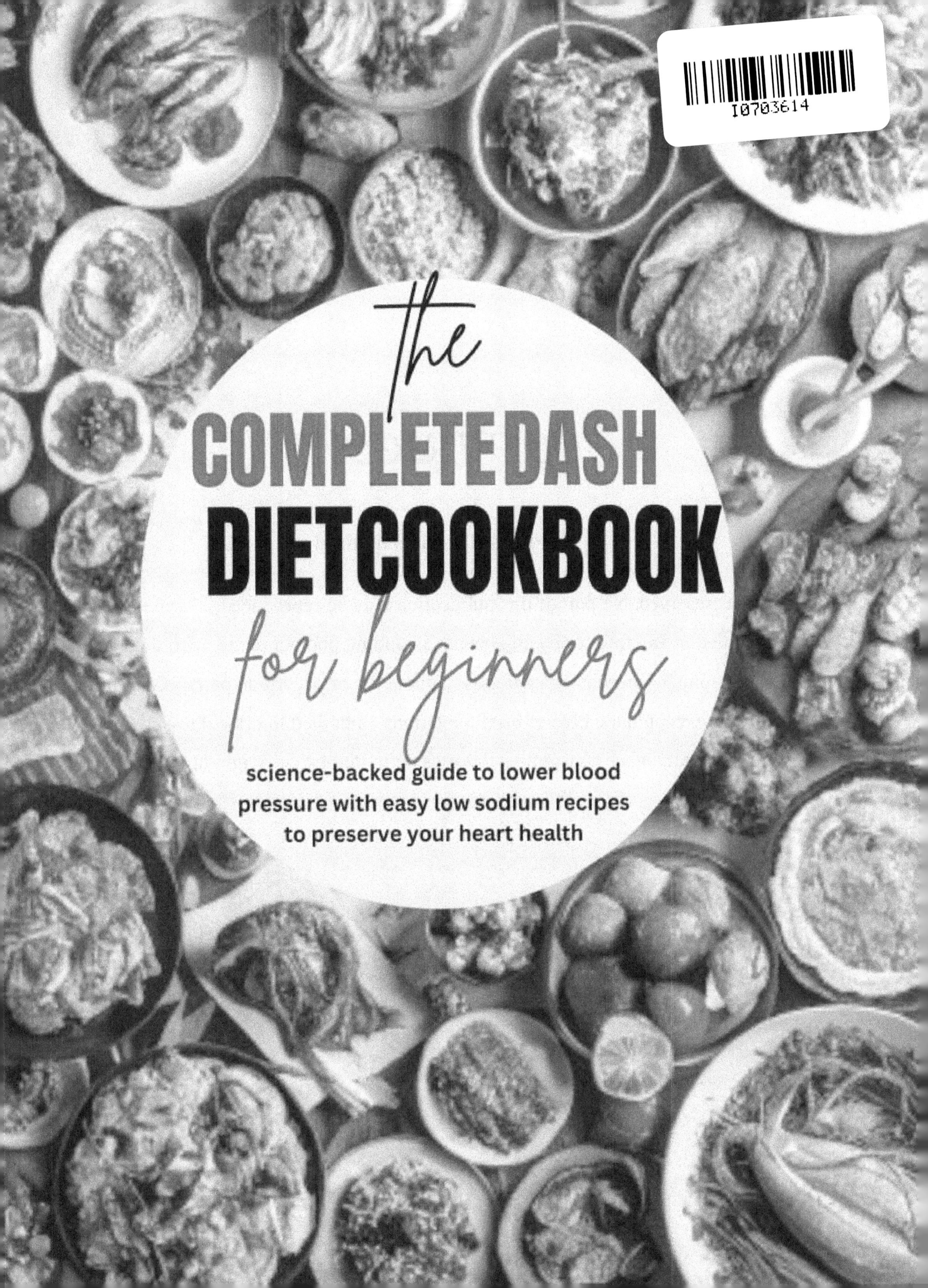

The
COMPLETE DASH
DIET COOKBOOK
for beginners
science-backed guide to lower blood pressure with easy low sodium recipes to preserve your heart health

# COPYRIGHT

# INTRODUCTION

The main objective of the Dietary Approaches to Stop Hypertension (DASH) diet is to treat hypertension, or high blood pressure. Blood pressure is a significant risk factor for heart disease, stroke, and other serious disorders. The DASH diet lowers sodium consumption and emphasizes complete foods that are high in minerals including potassium, calcium, magnesium, and fiber. It has been demonstrated by science that this combination can help lower blood pressure and enhance heart health in general.

I've witnessed the DASH diet's transformational impact as a professional health chef. Aria, one of my clients, was diagnosed with hypertension and was having difficulty controlling her condition without taking medicine. Aria's blood pressure significantly decreased, her energy levels increased, her sleep improved, and her general sense of well-being improved after implementing the DASH diet.

## Health Benefits of the DASH Diet

The DASH diet has numerous health advantages that can improve your quality of life and lower blood pressure.

**Reduce Blood Pressure:** One of the DASH diet's main goals is to lower blood pressure. A diet that emphasizes whole grains, fruits, vegetables, and lean proteins, and minimizes sodium intake can naturally lower blood pressure.

**Heart Health:** By lowering LDL cholesterol levels, the DASH diet not only lowers blood pressure but also improves heart health. Consequently, there is a decreased chance of heart disease and stroke.

**Weight management:** Eating more nutrient-dense, lower-calorie meals is encouraged by the DASH diet, which can aid in weight loss and help maintain a healthy weight. This is important since being overweight increases the chance of developing hypertension and other chronic illnesses.

**Diabetes Prevention and Management:** The DASH diet is a great option for preventing and controlling type 2 diabetes because it has a strong emphasis on whole grains, lean proteins, and healthy fats, which assist in managing blood sugar levels.

**Better Nutrient Intake:** Eating a wide range of fruits, vegetables, nuts, and seeds guarantees that you acquire several vital nutrients, such as fiber, potassium, calcium, and magnesium, all of which are critical for good health.

**Enhanced Mood and Energy:** Eating a well-balanced, whole-food-based diet can have a big impact on your mood and energy levels.

Following the DASH diet, many people claim to feel less moody and more energized.

# Essential DASH Diet Ingredients

Having the proper ingredients on hand is one of the keys to following the DASH diet successfully. The following are some staple foods that you should buy in bulk:

**Vegetables and fruits** should be the main components of your diet. To make sure you receive a wide range of nutrients, try to choose a colorful variety. Excellent options include fresh, frozen, and even canned food (without additional sugar or salt). Consider produce such as bell peppers, carrots, spinach, kale, bananas, berries, oranges, and apples.

**Whole Grains:** Rich in fiber and other nutrients, whole grains are an excellent source of nutrition. Include items in your meals such as barley, brown rice, quinoa, oats, and whole wheat pasta. These grains give you consistent energy throughout the day and aid in keeping you full.

**Lean Proteins:** Choose lean protein sources including tofu, beans, lentils, fish, poultry, and turkey. These proteins offer vital amino acids for muscle growth and repair and have a lower saturated fat content.

**Low-Fat Dairy:** Dairy products are a good way to get vitamin D and calcium. Select fat-free or low-fat dairy products like cheese, yogurt, and skim milk to maintain heart health and obtain these vital nutrients.

**Nuts and seeds** are a great source of fiber, protein, and good fats. Nuts like chia seeds, flaxseeds, walnuts, and almonds are excellent additions to your diet. Just watch the portion sizes, as they contain a lot of calories.

**Healthy Fats:** Include foods high in fat, such as avocado, and olive oil, and fatty fish like salmon. Heart health and general well-being depend on these fats.

**Herbs and Spices:** Keep a variety of herbs and spices on hand to add flavor to your food without consuming more sodium. Dried spices like paprika, cumin, and turmeric, together with fresh herbs like parsley, cilantro, and basil, can give your food more flavor and complexity.

# Kitchen Tools and Techniques

Having the proper kitchen gear and understanding a few essential cooking methods will make cooking DASH-friendly meals more fun and easier.

 To get you going, consider the following essential resources and advice:

**Sharp Knives:** For effective and secure food preparation, a decent set of sharp knives is needed. Purchase a serrated knife, paring knife, and chef's knife. It will be a lot simpler to chop fruits, vegetables, and meats if you keep them sharp.

**Cutting boards:** Use a variety of cutting boards to avoid contaminating raw meats with other foods. Choose easily cleaned boards made of plastic or wood.

**Blenders and food processors** are fantastic kitchen tools for swiftly cutting vegetables and creating soups, sauces, and smoothies. Moreover, a good blender can assist you in making nutrient-dense purees and smoothies.

**Steamer Basket:** Steam cooking preserves the nutrients found in veggies and is a healthful cooking technique. You may prepare a wide range of veggies, fish, and even dumplings without adding extra fat by using a steamer basket.

**Cookware that isn't stuck:** Cooking using non-stick cookware uses less oil, which makes it simpler to make meals that are lower in fat. Seek for sturdy, easily-cleanable, and premium non-stick cookware.

**A slow cooker or instant pot** are great kitchen tools for quickly and easily making nutritious meals. Soups, stews, and whole grains can be prepared without constant attention to detail.

**Measuring Cups and Spoons:** Following recipes correctly requires precise measurements, particularly when cutting sodium and managing portion sizes. To make sure you're adding the proper amounts of each ingredient, always have a set of measuring cups and spoons on hand.

**Salad Spinner:** Although washing and drying greens can be a laborious task, a salad spinner expedites and streamlines the procedure. Crisp, clean greens are essential for making tasty salads and avoiding soggy food.

# Cooking Methods

**Sautéing and stir-frying:** These methods swiftly cook vegetables, lean proteins, and grains while preserving their nutrients and flavors. They do this by using high heat and a tiny quantity of healthy oil. For optimal results, use a large skillet or a wok.

**Baking and roasting** are excellent ways to create tasty, evenly-cooked proteins and to bring out the natural sweetness of vegetables. Try roasting root veggies with your favorite herbs and a sprinkle of olive oil, such as carrots and sweet potatoes.

**Grilling:** Meats, veggies, and even fruits acquire a great smoky flavor from grilling. Additionally, because it lets extra fat escape from the dish, it's a healthful method of cooking. To improve flavor, experiment with marinades and use an outside barbecue or grill pan.

**Steaming:** As previously noted, steaming is an excellent fat-free method of cooking fish and vegetables. It maintains the food's moisture content and nutritional value.

**Blending and Pureeing:** To prepare soups, sauces, and smoothies, use a food processor or blender. When you want to create creamy textures without adding cream or butter, these tools are ideal.

# CHAPTER 1: MORNING MEALS

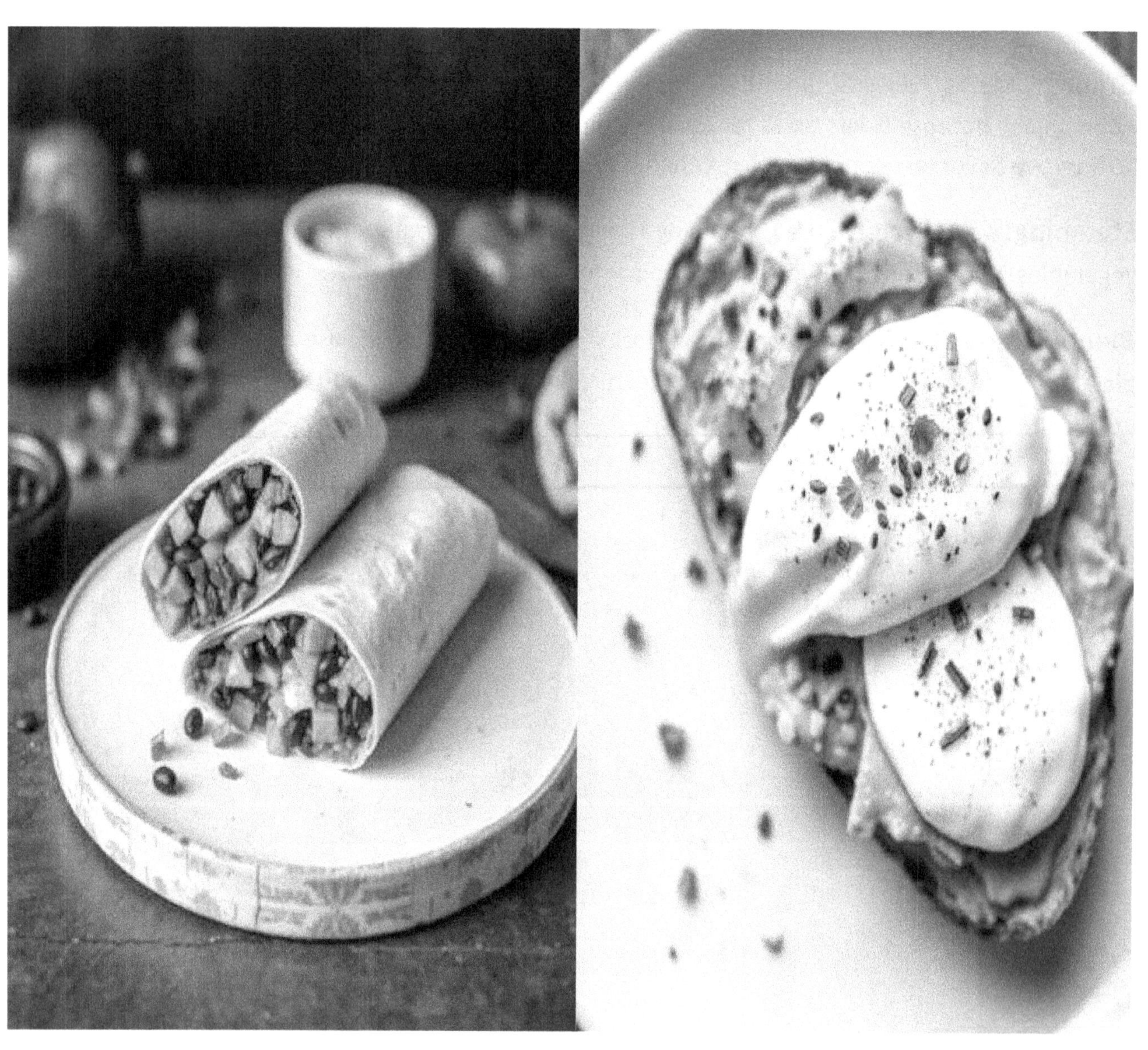

# Yogurt and Fresh Fruit Parfait

Serving: One

Prep Time: Half an hour

Cooking Time: - N/A

## Ingredients:

- One cup of Greek yogurt reduced in fat

- Half a cup of granola, ideally low in sugar

- Half a cup of freshly cut strawberries

- One-half cup of raw blueberries

- 1/2 cup chopped fresh kiwis

- One tablespoon honey, if desired

- One tablespoon of optional chia seeds

- Optional fresh mint leaves as a garnish

## How to Prepare:

### 1. Layer the Ingredients:

- ❖ Begin by filling a glass or bowl halfway with spoonfuls of Greek yogurt.
- ❖ Scatter some sliced strawberries on top.
- ❖ Scatter granola on top of the strawberries.
- ❖ Spread Greek yogurt on top once more.
- ❖ Add a layer of blueberries after that.
- ❖ Add a little extra granola.
- ❖ Spread Greek yogurt on top of the last layer.
- ❖ Sprinkle the leftover granola and chopped kiwis on top.

### 2. Incorporate Texture and Sweetness:

- ❖ If desired, drizzle honey over the upper layer to enhance sweetness.
- ❖ Add a little pinch of chia seeds for an additional fiber and omega-3 fatty acid boost (optional).

### 3. Garnish :

- ❖ Add a few fresh mint leaves for a flavorful burst of color at the end.

### 4. Serve:

- ❖ While the granola is crunchy, serve immediately. To preserve the texture of making ahead of time, keep the granola separate and add it only before serving.

## Ingredient Alternatives and Substitutes:

I. **Yogurt:** Use almond, soy, or coconut yogurt if you're lactose intolerant or would rather go plant-based.

II. **Granola:** For a variation in texture, replace granola with whole grain cereal or oats. Make sure you select low-sugar options to maintain compliance with your DASH diet.

III. **Fruits:** You can use whatever assortment of fresh fruits that you like or happen to have on hand. Bananas, mangoes, peaches, and berries are all great options.

IV. **Sweetener:** If you want a less sweet parfait, you can use agave syrup, or maple syrup, or eliminate the sweetener in place of the honey.

V. **Chia Seeds:** If preferred, you can eliminate or replace the chia seeds with flaxseeds.

## Nutritional Information:

- 300 calories
- 15g of protein
- 45g of carbohydrates
- 8g of dietary fiber
- 20g of sugars
- 8g of fat
- 2g of saturated fat
- 80 mg of sodium
- 450 mg of potassium
- 200 mg of calcium
- 70% of the Daily Value (DV) for vitamin C
- 15% of the DV for vitamin A
- 10% of the DV for iron

# Avocado Toast with Poached Egg

Serving: Two

Prep Time: Half an hour

Cooking Time: Half an hour

## Ingredients:

- One mature avocado

- Two whole grain pieces of bread

- Two big eggs

- One tablespoon white vinegar, salt, and pepper to taste, along with optional red pepper flakes

- Optional fresh lemon juice

- Optional fresh herb garnish

## How to Prepare:

**1. Prepare the Avocado:**

- ❖ Halve the avocado, take out the pit, and extract the flesh with a spoon.
- ❖ Mash the avocado in a bowl using a fork. Add a squeeze of fresh lemon juice and season with pepper and salt.

**2. Toast the Bread:**

- ❖ Toast the slices of whole grain bread until they are as crispy as you like.

## 3. Poach the Eggs:

- ❖ Add the white vinegar to a medium pot of water and bring it to a gentle simmer.
- ❖ Into a little bowl, crack each egg.
- ❖ Gently stir the water to form a vortex, then carefully place each egg in the center.
- ❖ Poach for three to four minutes, or until the yolks are still runny but the whites are set.
- ❖ Using a slotted spoon, remove the eggs and place them on paper towels to drain.

## 4. Assemble the Toast:

- ❖ Evenly spread the avocado mash over the slices of toasted bread.
- ❖ Top each piece with a poached egg.
- ❖ If preferred, add more salt, pepper, and red pepper flakes to the dish.
- ❖ Add fresh herbs as a garnish for an additional flavor boost.

## Ingredient Alternatives and Substitutes:

i. **Bread:** For a unique texture and flavor, use sourdough or gluten-free bread.

ii. **Eggs:** Hard-boiled, scrambled, or fried eggs can be used in place of poached eggs if desired.

iii. **Avocado:** Try it with hummus or a bean spread for a change.

## Nutritional Information:

- 300 calories
- 12g of protein
- 24g of carbohydrates
- 8g of dietary fiber
- 3g of sugars
- 18g of fat
- 3g of saturated fat
- 220 mg of sodium
- 700 mg of potassium
- 10% DV for vitamin A
- 15% DV for vitamin C
- Iron: 15% DV

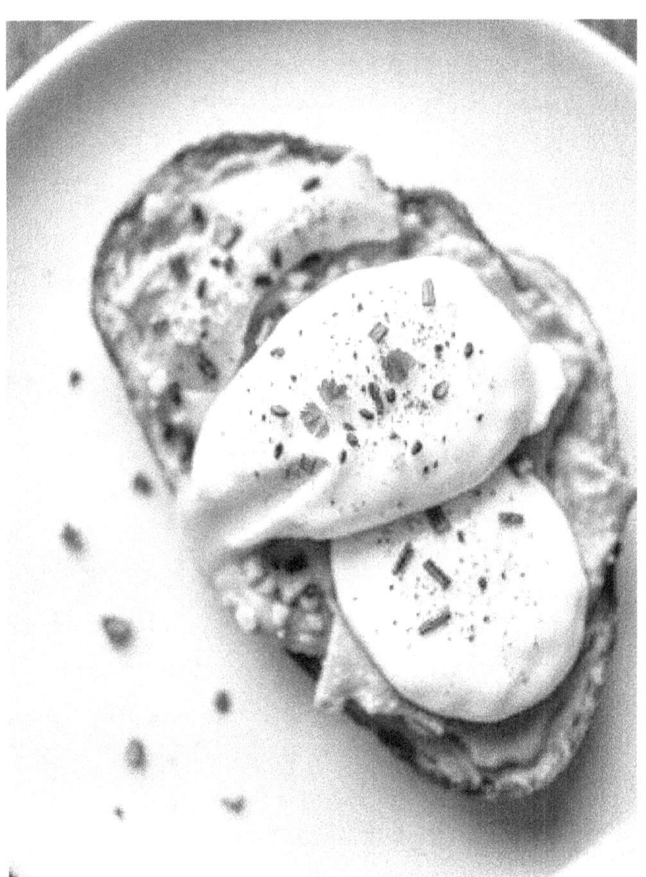

# Blueberry Oatmeal with Almonds

Serving: Two

Prep Time: Half an hour

Cooking Time: - Five minutes

## Ingredients:

- Two cups of water or low-fat milk

- One cup of old-fashioned oats

- A single cup of blueberries

- 1/4 cup of almonds, sliced

- One spoonful of honey or maple syrup

- One teaspoon of ground cinnamon

- A sprinkling of salt

- One-half teaspoon of extract from vanilla

## How to Prepare:

### 1. Cook the Oats:

- ❖ Boil the milk or water in a medium pot.
- ❖ When the oats are cooked and creamy, add the oats and a bit of salt, lower the heat, and simmer for approximately 5 minutes, stirring from time to time.

### 2. Incorporate Flavors:

- ❖ Mix in the vanilla extract and ground cinnamon.

### 3: Compile the oats

- ❖ Split the cooked oats into two portions.
- ❖ Place sliced almonds and fresh blueberries on top of each bowl.
- ❖ Drizzle with honey or maple syrup for sweetness.

## Ingredient Alternatives and Substitutes:

I. **Oats:** To achieve varying textures, use quick or steel-cut oats. Adapt the cooking time appropriately.

II. **Blueberries:** Feel free to use any other kind of berry, frozen or fresh.

III. **Almonds:** For a variation in crunch, try walnuts, pecans, or sunflower seeds.

## Nutritional Information:

- 350 calories
- 10g of protein
- 50g of carbohydrates
- 8g of dietary fiber
- 15g of sugars
- 12g of fat
- 1g of saturated fat
- 100 milligrams of sodium
- 400 milligrams of potassium
- Vitamin A: 2% Daily Value
- 10% DV for vitamin C
- Iron: 15% DV

# Spinach and Feta Omelette

Serving: One

Prep Time: Half an hour

Cooking Time: - Five minutes

## Ingredients:

- Three big eggs

- One cup of freshly chopped spinach

- 1/4 cup sliced tomatoes (optional)

- 1/4 cup crumbled feta cheese

- One tablespoon of butter or olive oil

- To taste, add salt and pepper.

## How to Prepare:

### 1. Get the Eggs Ready:

- ❖ Beat the eggs in a bowl with a dash of salt and pepper.

### 2. Cook the Spinach:

- ❖ Heat the butter or olive oil in a nonstick skillet over medium heat.
- ❖ Cook the chopped spinach for two minutes, or until it wilts.

### 3. Prepare the Omelette:

- ❖ Cover the spinach in the skillet with the beaten eggs.

- ❖ After letting the eggs set a little, gently lift the edges to allow the raw egg to flow beneath.
- ❖ When the eggs are almost set, top one side of the omelet with the diced tomatoes and feta cheese, if using.
- ❖ Once the omelet is entirely set, fold it in half and continue cooking for one to two minutes.

## Ingredient Alternatives and Substitutes:

I. **Eggs:** For a lower-cholesterol option, use egg whites or an egg substitute.

II. **Spinach:** For a different green, try kale or Swiss chard instead.

III. **Feta Cheese:** For a variation in flavor, use shredded mozzarella or goat cheese.

## Nutritional Information:

- 250 calories
- 18g of protein
- 4g of carbohydrates
- One gram of dietary fiber
- 2g of sugars
- 18g of fat
- 7g of saturated fat
- 350 mg of sodium
- 400 milligrams of potassium
- 40% DV for vitamin A
- 15% DV for vitamin C
- Iron: 15% DV

# Whole Wheat Pancakes with Berries

🍴 Serving: Four

⏱ Prep Time: 20 minutes

⏱ Cooking Time: - Half an hour

## Ingredients:

- One cup of whole wheat flour

- One tsp baking powder

- One cup low-fat milk

- One tablespoon sugar

- Half a teaspoon salt

- One big egg

- Two tablespoons of melted butter or olive oil

- One cup of mixed fresh berries, such as raspberries, blueberries, and strawberries; optional dish of honey or maple syrup

## How to Prepare:

### 1. Get the Batter Ready:

- ❖ Combine the whole wheat flour, baking powder, sugar, and salt in a sizable basin.
- ❖ Whisk the egg, milk, and melted butter or olive oil in a separate basin.
- ❖ Pour the wet ingredients into the dry ingredients, mixing just until combined.

### 2. Cook the Pancakes:

- ❖ Lightly oil or butter a nonstick skillet or griddle and heat it over medium heat.
- ❖ Fill the skillet with 1/4 cup of batter for each pancake.
- ❖ Cook for two to three minutes on each side, or until bubbles appear on the surface, then turn and continue cooking until the other side is golden brown.

### 3. Serve:

- ❖ Arrange the pancakes in a stack on a platter and garnish with the fresh berries.
- ❖ If preferred, drizzle with honey or maple syrup.

## Ingredient Alternatives and Substitutes:

I. **Flour:** For a gluten-free alternative, use a combination of flours without gluten.

II. **Milk:** Use soy, almond, or oat milk in its place.

III. **Berries:** Feel free to use any kind of fruit, frozen or fresh.

# Nutritional Information:

- 250 calories
- 8g of protein
- 40g of carbohydrates
- 6g of dietary fiber
- 8g of sugars
- 8g of fat
- 2g of saturated fat
- 450 mg of sodium
- 300 milligrams of potassium
- Vitamin A: 4% Daily Value
- 15% DV for vitamin C
- Iron: 15% D

# Chia Seed Pudding with Mango

Serving: Two

Prep Time: 4 hours of chilling

Cooking Time: - Five minutes

## Ingredients:

- One-fourth cup of chia seeds

- One cup of almond milk (or any other type of milk).

- One spoonful of honey or maple syrup

- One tsp of vanilla extract

- One cup of freshly diced mango

## How to Prepare:

### 1. Combine the Pudding:

- ❖ In a dish, mix almond milk, vanilla extract, honey or maple syrup, and chia seeds.
- ❖ Make sure the chia seeds are dispersed evenly by giving it a good stir.

### 2. Refrigerate:

- ❖ Once the mixture has thickened to a pudding-like consistency, cover and chill for at least 4 hours, or overnight.

### 3. Compose:

- ❖ Gently mix the chia seed pudding one more time to loosen up any lumps.
- ❖ Split the pudding between two jars or bowls.
- ❖ Add freshly chopped mango on top.

## Ingredient Alternatives and Substitutes:

I. **Milk:** Feel free to use conventional or plant-based milk.

II. **Sweetener:** For a less sweet pudding, substitute agave syrup or leave out the sweetener.

III. **Mango:** You can replace this with any other fresh fruit, such as peaches, blueberries, or strawberries.

## Nutritional Information:

- 250 calories
- Six grams of protein
- 35g of carbohydrates
- 10g of dietary fiber
- 20g of sugars
- 10g of fat
- 1g of saturated fat
- 100 milligrams of sodium
- 400 milligrams of potassium
- 15% DV for vitamin A
- 60% DV of vitamin C
- Iron: 15% DV

# Smoked Salmon and Cream Cheese Bagel

Serving: Two

Prep Time: Half an hour

Cooking Time: - N/A

## Ingredients:

- Four ounces of smoked salmon

- One split and toasted whole grain bagel

- Two tablespoons cream cheese (low-fat).

- 1/4 cup finely sliced red onion

- 1/4 cup capers

- Fresh dill for garnish

- Lemon wedges for serving

## How to Prepare:

### 1. Bagel Toasting

- ❖ Divide the whole grain bagel in half and toast it until it turns golden brown.

### 2. Assemble the Bagel:

- ❖ Evenly spread each half of the toasted bagel with the low-fat cream cheese.
- ❖ Top with pieces of smoked salmon.

❖ Add the capers and thinly sliced red onion.

## 3. Garnish and Serve:

❖ Arrange lemon wedges on the side and garnish with fresh dill.

## Ingredient Alternatives and Substitutes:

I. **Bagel:** Choose a whole wheat English muffin or a bagel without gluten.

II. **Cream Cheese**: Use Greek yogurt or a plant-based cream cheese substitute in its place.

III. **Smoked Salmon:** Use smoked trout or a substitute made of plants for smoked salmon.

## Nutritional Information:

- 300 calories
- 15g of protein
- 30g of carbohydrates
- 4g of dietary fiber
- 4g of sugars
- 12g of fat
- 4g of saturated fat
- 800 mg of sodium
- 300 milligrams of potassium
- Vitamin A: 6% Daily Value
- 10% DV for vitamin C
- Iron: 10% DV

# Sweet Potato and Black Bean Breakfast Burrito

Serving: One

Prep Time: 15 minutes

Cooking Time: - Half an hour

## Ingredients:

- One medium sweet potato, chopped and peeled

- Half a cup of rinsed and drained black beans

- Two large eggs

- 1/4 cup of shredded cheddar cheese

- 2 whole wheat tortillas

- One tablespoon olive oil

- 1/4 cup salsa

- Season with salt and pepper

- Garnish with fresh cilantro, if desired

## How to Prepare:

### 1. Prepare the Sweet Potatoes:

❖ In a skillet over medium heat, warm the olive oil.

❖ Add the diced sweet potatoes and simmer for about ten minutes, or until they are soft and starting to color.

❖ Add pepper and salt for seasoning.

## 2. Get the Eggs Ready:

❖ Beat the eggs in a bowl with a dash of pepper and salt.
❖ Scramble the eggs in the skillet containing the sweet potatoes until they are thoroughly done.

## 3. Compose the Burritos:

❖ Spread the sweet potato and egg mixture equally among the flattened tortillas.
❖ Include the salsa, shredded cheddar cheese, and black beans.
❖ To make burritos, roll the tortillas.

## 4. Serve:

❖ If wanted, garnish with fresh cilantro and serve right away.

## Ingredient Alternatives and Substitutes:

- **Tortillas:** For a gluten-free substitute, use corn tortillas.
- **Cheese:** If necessary, use dairy-free cheese in its place.
- **Beans:** As an alternative, use kidney or pinto beans.

## Nutritional Information:

- 400 calories
- 18g of protein
- 50g of carbohydrates
- 10g of dietary fiber
- 6g of sugars
- 15g of fat
- 4g of saturated fat
- 600 mg of sodium
- 700 mg of potassium
- 120% DV of vitamin A
- 20% DV for vitamin C
- Iron: 15% DV

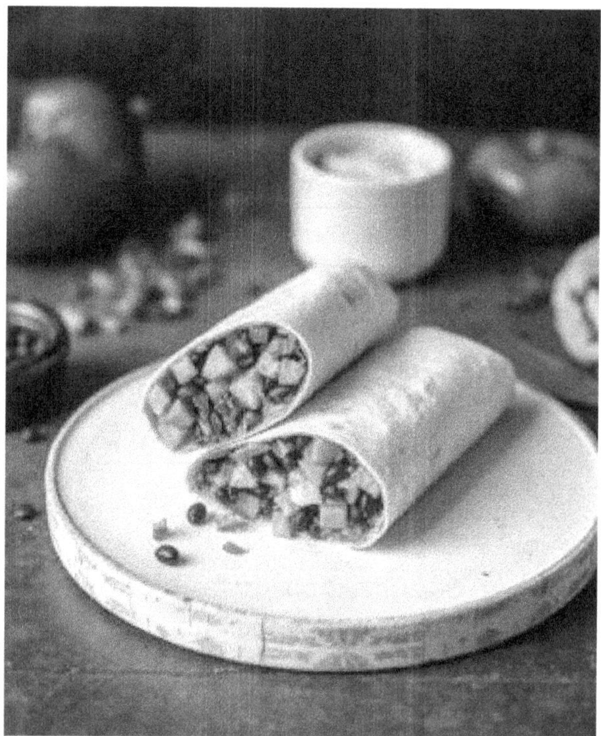

# Apple Cinnamon Quinoa

Serving: Two

Prep Time: 20 minutes

Cooking Time: - Half an hour

## Ingredients:

- One cup of washed quino

- Two cups of water or nonfat milk

- 1/4 cup raisins

- 1 peeled, cored, and chopped apple

- One spoonful of honey or maple syrup

- One teaspoon of ground cinnamon

- 1/4 cup of chopped walnuts

- 1/2 teaspoon of vanilla extract

- A dash of salt

## How to Prepare:

### 1. Prepare the Quinoa:

- ❖ Heat milk or water in a medium pot until it boils.
- ❖ Once the quinoa is soft and the liquid has been absorbed, add a pinch of salt, lower the heat, and simmer the quinoa for about fifteen minutes.

### 2. Incorporate Flavors

- ❖ Mix in the chopped apple, raisins, ground cinnamon, honey or maple syrup, and vanilla essence.
- ❖ Cook until the apple is soft, about 5 more minutes.

### 3. Serve :

- ❖ Spoon the quinoa mixture into dishes; sprinkle chopped walnuts over top.

## Ingredient Alternatives and Substitutes:

I. **Quinoa:** Use farro or steel-cut oats in place of.
II. **Milk:** For a dairy-free option, use oat, soy, or almond milk.
III. **Walnuts:** You can use sunflower seeds, pecans, or almonds.

## Nutritional Information:

- 350 calories
- 10g of protein
- 60g of carbohydrates
- 8g of dietary fiber
- 20g of sugars
- 10g of fat
- 1g of saturated fat
- 100 milligrams of sodium
- 500 milligrams of potassium
- Vitamin A: 2% Daily Value
- Vitamin C: 8% Daily Value
- Iron: 20% DV

# Greek Yogurt with Honey and Walnuts

Serving: Two

Prep Time: Five minutes

Cooking Time: - N/A

## Ingredients:

- One cup of Greek yogurt reduced in fat

- 1/4 cup of walnuts, chopped

- Two tsp honey

- Optional fresh mint leaves as a garnish

## How to Prepare:

### 1. Get the Yogurt Ready:

- ❖ Transfer the Greek yogurt into a bowl using a spoon.

### 2. Incorporate Honey and Walnuts:

- ❖ Pour honey onto the yogurt.
- ❖ Garnish with chopped walnuts.

### 3. Garnish:

- ❖ If preferred, add some fresh mint leaves for a cool touch.

## Ingredient Alternatives and Substitutes:

I. **Yogurt:** For a dairy-free option, use coconut, soy, or almond yogurt.
II. **Honey:** Use agave nectar or maple syrup in place of.
III. **Walnuts**: Sunflower seeds, almonds, or pecans can be used.

## Nutritional Information:

I. 300 calories
II. 15g of protein
III. 35g of carbohydrates
IV. 2g of dietary fiber
V. 25g of sugars
VI. 12g of fat
VII. 2g of saturated fat
VIII. 100 milligrams of sodium
IX. 300 milligrams of potassium
X. Vitamin A: 2% Daily Value
XI. Vitamin C: 2% Daily Value
XII. Iron: 6% DV

# Chapter 2: Drinks and Smoothies

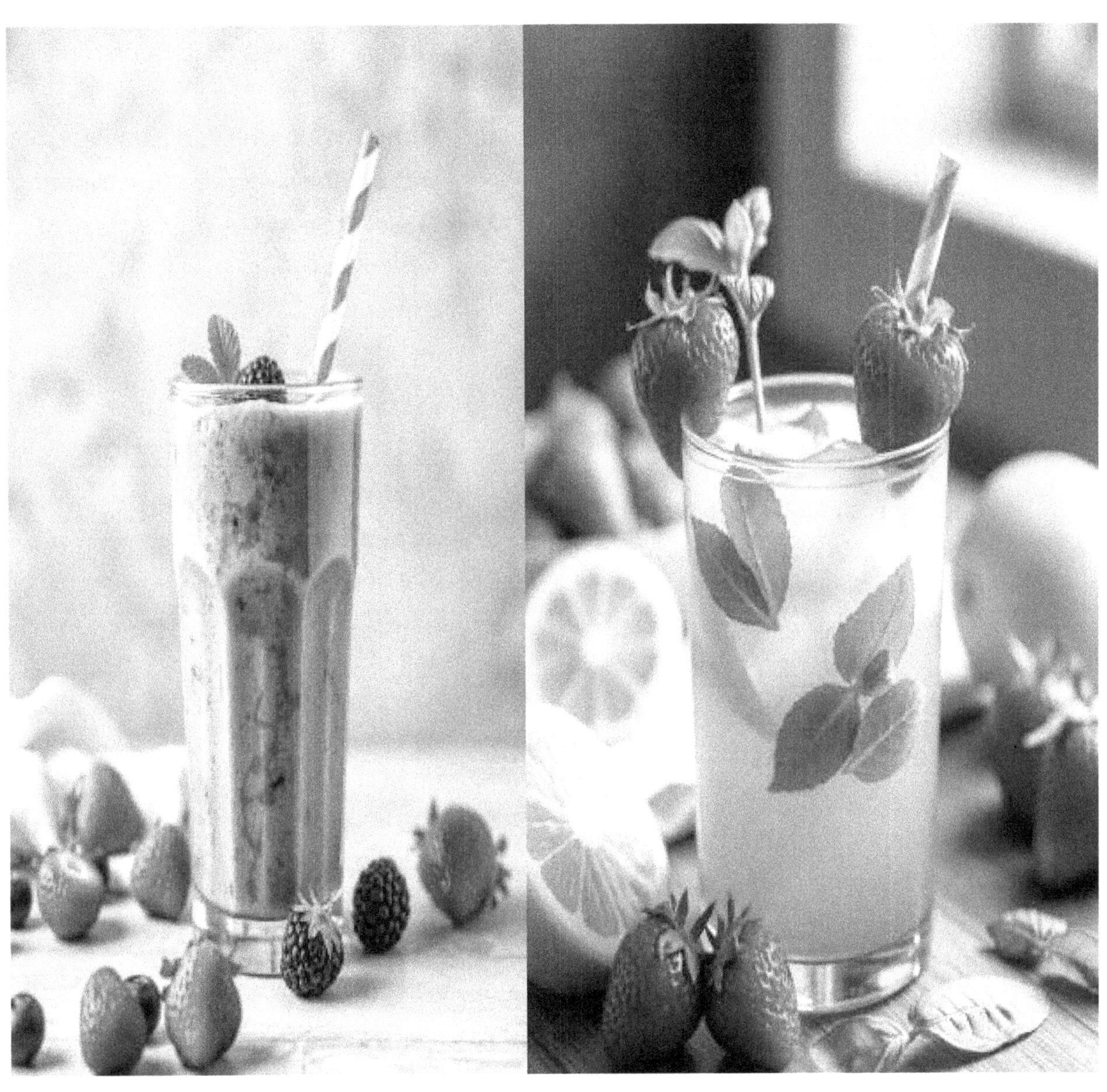

# Green Detox Smoothie

Serving: One

Prep Time: 20 minutes

Cooking Time: Five minutes

## Ingredients:

- One cup of de-stemmed kale leaves
- half a cup of spinach leaves
- half a banana
- one-half apple, peeled and diced
- half a cucumber, sliced and peeled
- One tablespoon of newly squeezed lemon juice
- one cup of coconut water or water
- One teaspoon of optional chia seeds
- Cubes of ice (optional)

## How to Prepare:

### 1. Mix the ingredients:

- ❖ In a blender, add the kale, spinach, banana, apple, cucumber, lemon juice, and water.
- ❖ Process till smooth.
- ❖ If desired, add ice cubes and mix once more until smooth.

### 2. Serve:

- ❖ Pour into a glass and start sipping right away.
- ❖ If using, top with a sprinkle of chia seeds.

## Ingredient Alternatives and Substitutes:

I. **Kale:** Use collard greens or Swiss chard.
II. Change out the spinach with romaine lettuce.
III. **Banana:** To achieve creaminess without the sweetness, use avocado.
IV. **Green tea** can be used instead of water to increase the antioxidant content.

## Nutritional Information:

- 150 calories
- 3g of protein
- 35g of carbohydrates
- 8g of dietary fiber
- 15g of sugars
- Fat: 1 gram
- 0g of saturated fat
- 50 milligrams of sodium
- 700 milligrams of potassium
- 150% DV of vitamin A
- Vitamin C: 100% DV
- 15% iron DV

# Berry Blast Smoothie

Serving: Two

Prep Time: 20 minutes

Cooking Time:

Five minutes

## Ingredients:

- One cup of mixed berries, including raspberries, blueberries, and strawberries
- half a cup of Greek yogurt
- half a banana
- One spoonful of maple syrup or honey
- One cup of almond milk
- Cubes of ice (optional)

## How to Prepare:

### 1. Mix the ingredients:

- ❖ In a blender, combine berries, Greek yogurt, banana, honey, and almond milk.
- ❖ Process till smooth.
- ❖ If desired, add ice cubes and mix once more until smooth.

### 2. Serve:

- ❖ Transfer into a glass and immediately begin to drink.

## Ingredient Alternatives and Substitutes:

I. **Berries:** Feel free to combine frozen or fresh berries.
II. **Greek yogurt:** For a dairy-free option, use plant-based yogurt in its place.
III. Use any milk to make almond milk.
IV. **Serving:** There is one serving per recipe.

## Nutritional Information:

- 200 calories
- 8g of protein
- 38g of carbohydrates
- 6g of dietary fiber
- 22g of sugars
- 4g of fat
- 0g of saturated fat
- 100 milligrams of sodium
- 500 milligrams of potassium
- 4% DV of vitamin A
- Vitamin C: Completely DV
- Iron: 8% DV

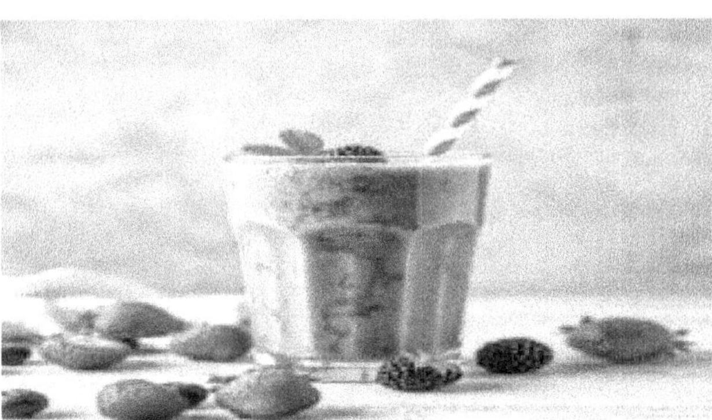

# Tropical Paradise Smoothie

Serving: one

Prep Time: 20 minutes

Cooking Time: Five minutes

## Ingredients:

- One cup of frozen pineapple chunks

- Half a cup of frozen mango chunks

- half a banana

- half a cup of coconut milk

- half a cup of orange juice

- One tablespoon of coconut shreds (optional)

- Cubes of ice (optional)

## How to Prepare:

### 1. Mix the ingredients:

- ❖ In a blender, combine the pineapple, mango, banana, coconut milk, and orange juice.
- ❖ Process till smooth.
- ❖ If desired, add ice cubes and mix once more until smooth.

### 2. Serve:

- ❖ Pour into a glass and start sipping right away.
- ❖ If used, scatter the shredded coconut on top.

## Ingredient Alternatives and Substitutes:

I. **Pineapple:** Try frozen papaya or peaches instead.

II. **Mango:** Use frozen apricots or peaches in place of the mango.

III. **Coconut Milk:** To have a distinct flavor, use soy or almond milk.

IV. Use apple or pineapple juice for your orange juice

## Nutritional Information:

- 250 calories
- 3g of protein
- 55g of carbohydrates
- 6g of dietary fiber
- 45g of sugar and 5g of fat
- Four grams of saturated fat
- 40 milligrams of sodium
- 700 milligrams of potassium
- 15% DV for vitamin A
- 200% DV for vitamin C
- 10% DV for iron

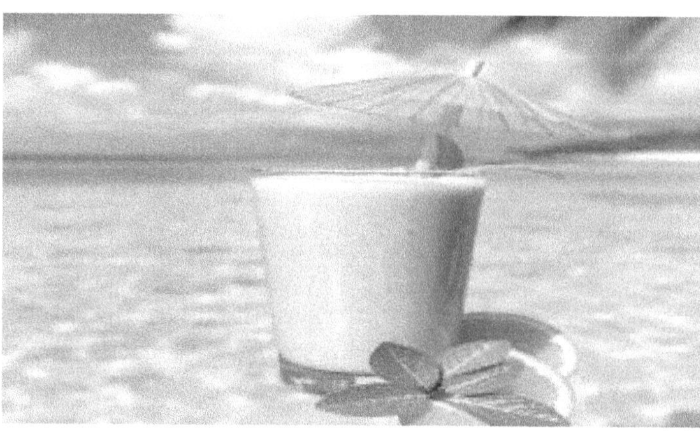

# Almond Butter and Banana Smoothie

Serving: One

Prep Time: 20 minutes

Cooking Time: Five minutes

## Ingredients:

- One banana
- One spoonful of butter made of almonds
- One cup of almond milk
- One tsp honey or maple syrup
- 1/4 tsp ground cinnamon
- Cubes of ice (optional)

## How to Prepare:

### 1. Mix the ingredients:

- ❖ In a blender, combine the banana, ground cinnamon, almond butter, almond milk, and honey.
- ❖ Process till smooth.
- ❖ If desired, add ice cubes and mix once more until smooth.

### 2. Serve:

- ❖ Pour into a glass and start sipping right away.

## Ingredient Alternatives and Substitutes:

I. **Banana:** For richness with less sugar, use avocado instead of banana.

II. **Almond butter** can be substituted with peanut butter or sunflower seed butter.

III. Use any kind of milk to make almond milk

## Nutritional Information:

- 250 calories
- 5g of protein
- 40g of carbohydrates
- 5g of dietary fiber
- 25g of sugars
- 9g of fat
- One gram of saturated fat
- 150 milligrams of sodium
- 600 milligrams of potassium
- Vitamin A: 2% Daily Value
- 15% DV for vitamin C
- Iron: 6% DV

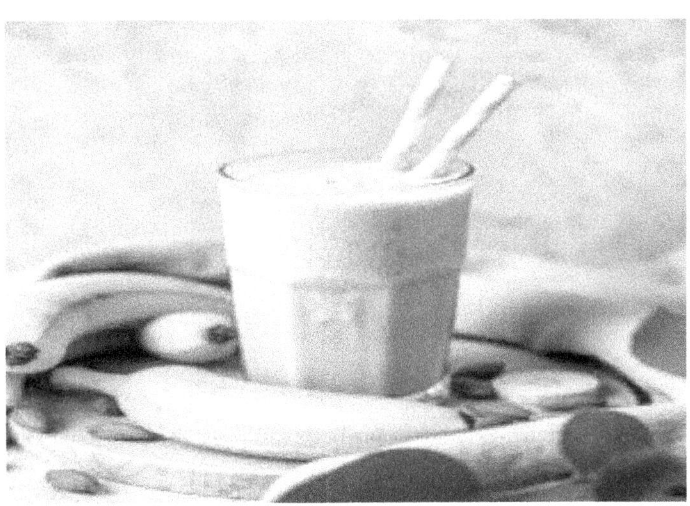

# Refreshing Cucumber Mint Water

Serving: Eight

Prep Time: 20 minutes

Cooking Time: Five minutes

## Ingredients:

- One cucumber cut thinly

- one-fourth cup of fresh mint leaves

- Eight glasses of water

- Cubes of ice (optional)

## How to Prepare:

### 1. Mix the Ingredients:

- ❖ Mint leaves and cucumber slices should be combined in a big pitcher.
- ❖ Stir thoroughly after adding the water.
- ❖ Give it a minimum of one hour to settle so the flavors can fully integrate.

### 2. Serve:

- ❖ If desired, pour into glasses over ice cubes.

## Ingredient Alternatives and Substitutes:

I. Use thinly sliced lime or lemon for the cucumber.

II. For a distinct flavor, try substituting rosemary or basil for the mint.

## Nutritional Information:

- Five calories
- Glycogen: 1g; Protein: 0g
- 0 grams of dietary fiber
- Sugar content: 0g
- Fat: 0 grams
- 0g of saturated fat
- Ten milligrams of sodium
- 50 milligrams of potassium
- Vitamin A: 2% Daily Value
- Vitamin C: 4% Daily Value
- Iron: 2% DV

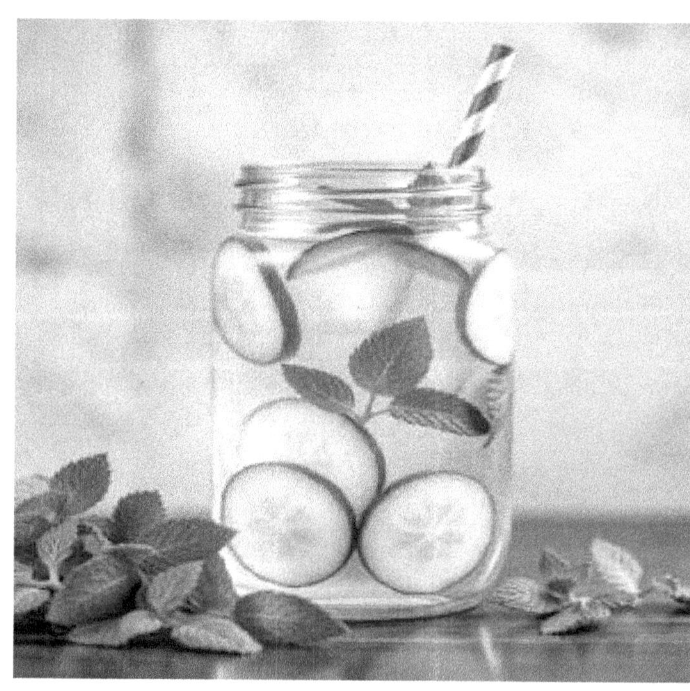

# Classic Tomato Juice

Serving: Two

Prep Time: Ten minute

Cooking Time: Half an hour

## Ingredients:

- Four big, ripe tomatoes, diced
- one-fourth cup water
- 1/4 tsp salt
- 1/4 tsp black pepper
- One tablespoon of lemon juice
- Garnish with fresh basil leaves (optional).

## How to Prepare:

### 1. Mix the ingredients:

- ❖ In a blender, combine tomatoes, water, salt, and black pepper.
- ❖ Process till smooth.
- ❖ To get rid of the pulp, strain the mixture through a fine screen.

### 2. Incorporate Lemon Juice:

- ❖ Add the lemon juice and stir.

### 3. Serve:

- ❖ Transfer into glasses and, if you like, decorate with fresh basil leaves.

## Ingredient Alternatives and Substitutes:

I. **Tomatoes:** If fresh tomatoes are unavailable, use canned tomatoes instead.
II. **Lemon juice** can be substituted with lime juice.

## Nutritional Information:

- 50 calories
- 2g of protein
- 12g of carbohydrates
- 3 grams of dietary fiber
- 7g of sugars
- Fat: 0 grams
- 0g of saturated fat
- 150 milligrams of sodium
- 500 milligrams of potassium
- 20% DV for vitamin A
- 60% of vitamin C DV
- Iron: 4% DV

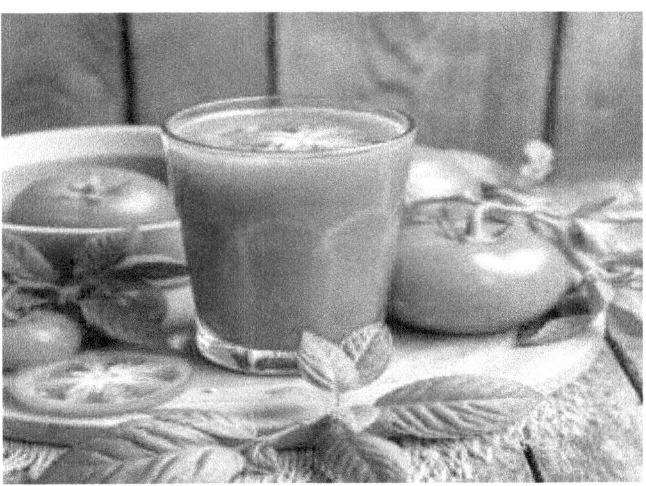

# Herbal Iced Tea

Serving: Two

Prep Time: Ten minutes

Cooking Time: Half an hour

## Ingredients:

- Four herbal tea bags (you can choose between chamomile and peppermint).
- Boil 4 cups of water.
- One tablespoon of maple syrup or honey (optional)
- Slices of lemon are optional as a garnish.
- Garnish with fresh mint leaves (optional).
- Cubes of ice

## How to Prepare:

### 1. Prepare the Tea:

- ❖ Tir the tea bags into a heat-resistant pitcher.
- ❖ Cover tea bags with boiling water.
- ❖ After five minutes of steeping, take out the tea bags.

### 2. Chill and sweeten:

- ❖ If preferred, stir in honey or maple syrup.
- ❖ After allowing the tea to reach room temperature, chill it in the refrigerator.

### 3. Serve:

- ❖ If preferred, garnish with lemon slices and mint leaves and serve over ice cubes.

## Ingredient Alternatives and Substitutes:

I. Use any flavor of herbal tea in the herbal tea bags.

II. **Sweetener:** For a reduced calorie option, omit or use stevia.

III. **Servings:** There are four servings per recipe.

IV.

## Nutritional Information:

- Five calories
- Protein: nil
- One gram of carbohydrates
- 0 grams of dietary fiber
- 1g of sugars
- Fat: 0 grams
- 0g of saturated fat
- Sodium: 0 mg
- 20 milligrams of potassium
- Vitamin A: 0% DV
- Vitamin C: 2% DV
- Iron: 0% DV

# Warm Turmeric Golden Milk

Serving: One

Prep Time: 20 minutes

Cooking Time: Five minutes

## Ingredients:

- One cup of milk, any kind of milk will do
- half a teaspoon of turmeric powder
- 1/4 tsp ground cinnamon
- 1/4 tsp ground ginger
- One spoonful of maple syrup or honey
- A dash of dark pepper

## How to Prepare:

### 1. Warm up the milk:

- ❖ Almond milk should be heated in a small saucepan over medium heat without boiling.

### 2. Add the sweetener and spices:

- ❖ Add the ginger, cinnamon, turmeric, honey, and black pepper and stir.
- ❖ Stir continuously and heat gently for an additional two minutes.

### 3. Serve:

- ❖ Transfer into a cup and savor it warm.

## Ingredient Alternatives and Substitutes:

Use any milk to make almond milk.

**Honey:** You can use maple syrup or agave nectar in its place.

**Spices:** Use a pre-mixed combination of turmeric lattes or adjust the spices to your taste.

## Nutritional Information:

- 150 calories
- 2g of protein
- 25g of carbohydrates
- One gram of dietary fiber
- 20g of sugars
- 5g of fat
- 0g of saturated fat
- 150 milligrams of sodium
- 200 milligrams of potassium
- 10% DV for vitamin A
- Vitamin C: 2% Daily Value
- Iron: 6% DV

# Citrus Infused Water

Serving: Eight

Prep Time: 20 minutes

Cooking Time: Five minutes

## Ingredients:

- One thinly sliced lemon
- one thinly sliced lime
- one thinly sliced orange, and eight cups of water
- Cubes of ice

## How to Prepare:

### 1. Mix the Ingredients:

- ❖ Slices of orange, lime, and lemon should be combined in a big pitcher.
- ❖ Stir thoroughly after adding the water.

### 2. Cool and Present:

- ❖ To let the flavors settle in, refrigerate for at least an hour.
- ❖ Over ice cubes, serve.

## Ingredient Alternatives and Substitutes:

I. Use any combination of citrus fruits, for as tangerines or grapefruits.

II. **Water:** For a bubbly variation, use sparkling water.

## Nutritional Information:

- Five calories
- Protein: nil
- One gram of carbohydrates
- 0 grams of dietary fiber
- Sugar content: 0g
- Fat: 0 grams
- 0g of saturated fat
- Sodium: 0 mg
- 10 milligrams of potassium
- Vitamin A: 2% Daily Value
- 10% of vitamin C DV
- Iron: 0% DV

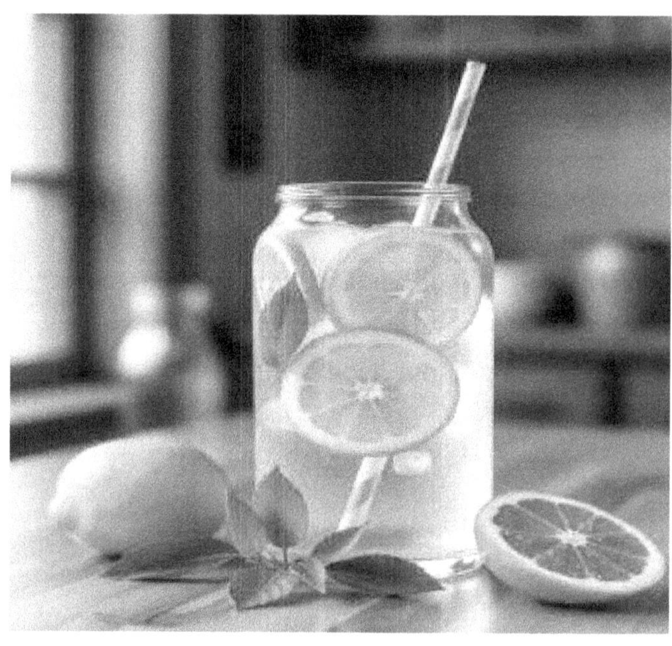

# Strawberry Basil Lemonade

Serving: four

Prep Time: 20 minutes

Cooking Time: Ten minutes

## Ingredients:

- One cup of recently hulled and chopped strawberries
- half a cup of fresh basil leaves
- one-half cup of freshly squeezed lemon juice
- 1/4 cup agave syrup or honey
- two cups of water
- Cubes of ice

## How to Prepare:

### 1. Mix the ingredients:

- ❖ Blend strawberries, basil leaves, honey, lemon juice, and one cup of water in a blender.
- ❖ Process till smooth.

### 2. Mix and strain:

- ❖ The mixture should be strained into a pitcher using a fine strainer.
- ❖ After adding the final cup of water, thoroughly stir.

### 3. Serve:

- ❖ Pour over ice cubes in glasses.

## Ingredient Alternatives and Substitutes:

I. Swap out the strawberries for raspberries or blueberries.
II. Replace basil with thyme or mint.
III. Honey: Replace sugar with stevia.

## Nutritional Information:

- 80 calories
- 1g of protein
- 20g of carbohydrates
- dietary fiber: two grams
- 18g of sugars
- Fat: 0 grams
- 0g of saturated fat
- Sodium: 0 mg
- 150 milligrams of potassium
- Vitamin A: 2% Daily Value
- 60% DV for vitamin C
- Iron: 2% DV

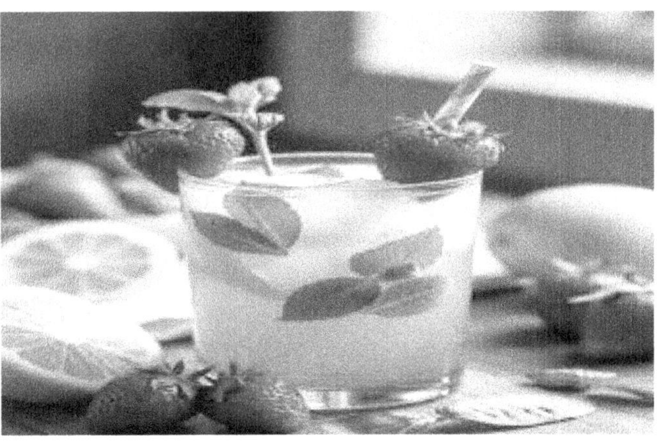

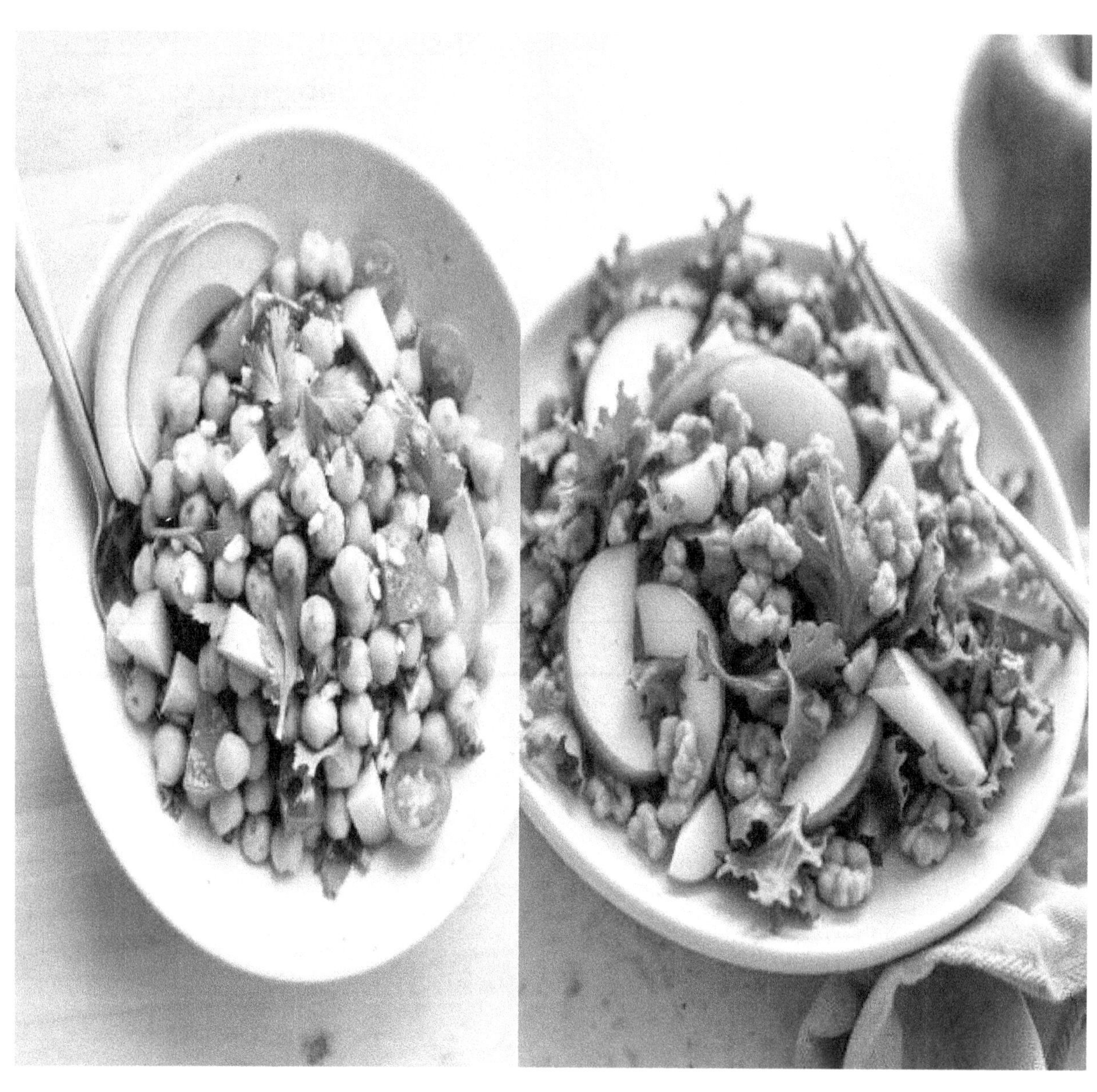

# Quinoa and Black Bean Salad

Serving: four

Prep Time: Twenty minutes

Cooking Time: 15 minutes

## Ingredients:

- One cup of quinoa
- Half a cup of water
- One cup of cooked black beans (homemade or from a can).
- One sliced red bell pepper
- Half a cup of corn kernels, frozen or fresh
- 1/4 cup coarsely chopped red onion
- 1/4 cup finely chopped fresh cilantro
- Juiced one lime
- Two tsp olive oil
- To taste, add salt and black pepper.

## How to Prepare:

### 1. Prepare the Quinoa:

- ❖ Clean the quinoa with cool water.
- ❖ Put the quinoa and water in a medium-sized saucepan. Reduce heat after bringing it to a boil.
- ❖ Once the quinoa is soft and the water has been absorbed, cover it and cook it for around 15 minutes—fluff with a fork and set aside to cool.

### 2. Get the Salad Ready:

- ❖ Combine cooked quinoa, black beans, corn, red onion, cilantro, and bell pepper in a big bowl.
- ❖ Combine lime juice, olive oil, salt, and pepper in a small bowl.
- ❖ Drizzle the salad with the dressing and toss to coat.

### 3. Provide:

- ❖ It can be served at room temperature or chilled.

## Ingredient Alternatives and Substitutes:

I.  **Quinoa:** Replace with bulgur or cooked farro.
II.  **Black Beans**: Use chickpeas or kidney beans.
III.  **Corn:** For a variation in texture, use cooked edamame.

## Nutritional Information:

- 250 calories
- 9g of protein
- 45g of carbohydrates
- 8g of dietary fiber
- 4g of sugars
- 7g of fat
- 1g of saturated fat
- 200 milligrams of sodium
- 500 milligrams of potassium
- 20% DV for vitamin A
- 30% DV for vitamin C
- Iron: 15% DV

# Greek Salad with Feta

Serving: four

Prep Time: N/B

Cooking Time: Ten minutes

## Ingredients:

- Two cups of halved cherry tomatoes
- One diced cucumber
- Half a red onion, cut thinly
- 1/2 cup pitted Kalamata olives
- 1/2 cup of feta cheese, crumbled
- Fourteen ounces of virgin olive oil
– Two tsp red wine vinegar.
- One teaspoon of oregano, dried
- To taste, add salt and black pepper.

## How to Prepare:

### 1. Mix the Vegetables:

❖ Combine cherry tomatoes, cucumber, red onion, olives, and feta cheese in a sizable bowl.

### 2. Get the Dressing Ready:

❖ Combine the olive oil, red wine vinegar, oregano, salt, and pepper in a small bowl.

### 3. Discard and Present:

❖ Drizzle the salad with the dressing and gently toss to mix.

❖ Refrigerate or serve immediately when ready to serve.

## Ingredient Alternatives and Substitutes:

I. **Feta Cheese:** Use goat cheese or a substitute cheese that doesn't contain dairy.

II. **Karama Olives:** Replace with capers or green olives.

## Nutritional Information:

- 220 calories
- 8g of protein
- 15g of carbohydrates
- 3g of dietary fiber
- 4g of sugars
- 16g of fat
- 5g of saturated fat
- 600 mg of sodium
- 350 milligrams of potassium
- 15% DV for vitamin A
- 25% DV for vitamin C
- Iron: 10% DV

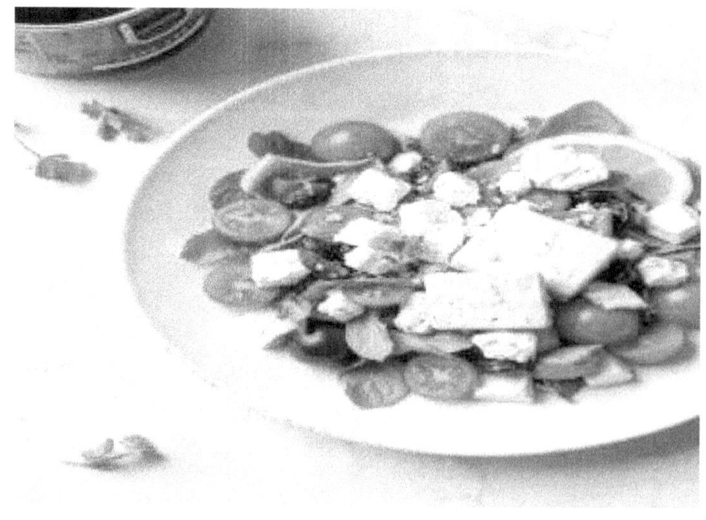

# Roasted Beet and Orange Salad

Serving: four

Prep Time: N/B

Cooking Time: Ten minutes

## Ingredients:

- Four medium beets, sliced into wedges after peeling.
- Two tsp olive oil
- To taste, add salt and black pepper.
- Two peeled and segmented oranges
- 1/4 cup of goat cheese, crumbled
- 1/4 cup of walnuts, chopped
- Two tsp balsamic vinegar
- One tablespoon of honey

## How to Prepare:

### 1. Grill the Beetroots:

- ❖ Set oven temperature to 200°C/400°F.
- ❖ Combine salt, pepper, and olive oil with the beet slices.
- ❖ Arrange them on a baking sheet, then roast them for 35 to 40 minutes, or until they become soft. Allow to cool.

### 2. Get the Salad Ready:

- ❖ Combine the goat cheese, walnuts, orange segments, and roasted beets in a big bowl.

### 3. Get the Dressing Ready:

- ❖ Combine honey and balsamic vinegar in a small basin.

### 4. Provide:

- ❖ Pour the dressing over the salad and give it a little stir.
- ❖ Present right away.

## Ingredient Alternatives and Substitutes:

I. **Beets:** For a variation in taste, use roasted sweet potatoes.

II. **Goat Cheese:** For a dairy-free option, replace with feta cheese or remove.

III. **Apples or pears** can be substituted for oranges for a unique flavor.

## Nutritional Information:

- 220 calories
- Six grams of protein
- 28g of carbohydrates
- 6g of dietary fiber
- 15g of sugars
- 11g of fat
- 3g of saturated fat
- 150 milligrams of sodium
- 500 milligrams of potassium
- 20% DV for vitamin A
- 60% DV of vitamin C
- Iron: 10% DV

# Kale and Apple Salad with Walnuts

Serving: four

Prep Time: 20 minutes

Cooking Time: Ten minutes

## Ingredients:

- 4 cups chopped and stem-free kale
- One cored and finely sliced apple
- 1/4 cup roasted walnuts
- 1/4 cup of feta cheese, crumbled
- Two tsp olive oil
- One tsp of apple cider vinegar
- One tablespoon of honey
- To taste, add salt and black pepper.

## How to Prepare:

1. **Get the Kale Ready:**
   - ❖ To soften the leaves, massage the kale for one to two minutes with a small amount of olive oil and salt.

2. **Get the Salad Ready:**
   - ❖ Combine feta cheese, walnuts, apple slices, and kale in a big bowl.

3. **Get the Dressing Ready:**
   - ❖ Combine olive oil, honey, apple cider vinegar, salt, and pepper in a small bowl.

4. **Provide:**
   - ❖ Drizzle the salad with the dressing and mix thoroughly.

- ❖ Present right away.

## Ingredient Alternatives and Substitutes:

- ❖ **Kale:** Replace with Swiss chard or spinach.
- ❖ **Apple:** Cut up pieces of orange or pear.
- ❖ **Feta Cheese:** Omit or replace with goat cheese.

## Nutritional Information:

- 180 calories
- Six grams of protein
- 20g of carbohydrates
- 4g of dietary fiber
- 12g of sugars
- 10g of fat
- 2g of saturated fat
- 200 milligrams of sodium
- 400 milligrams of potassium
- 25% DV for vitamin A
- 30% DV for vitamin C
- Iron: 8% DV

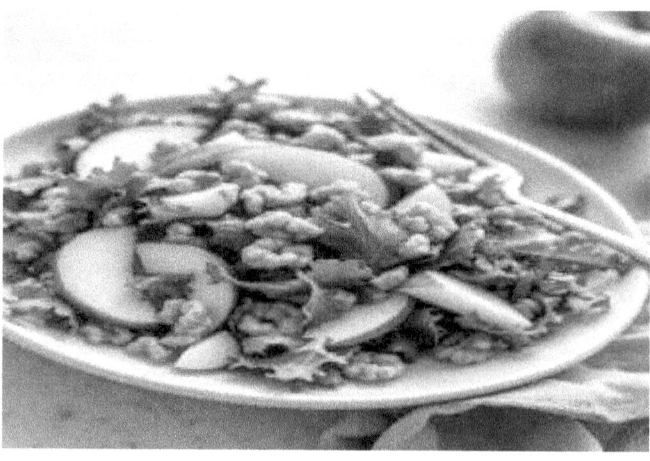

# Classic Caesar Salad with a DASH Twist

Serving: four

Prep Time: N/B

Cooking Time: Ten minutes

## Ingredients:

- Four cups chopped romaine lettuce
- A half cup of Parmesan cheese, shaved
- One-half cup of whole-wheat crisps
- One-fourth cup of Greek yogurt
- Half a cup of lemon juice
- One tablespoon of mustard dijon
- One minced garlic clove
- One tablespoon of olive oil
- To taste, add salt and black pepper.

## How to Prepare:

1. **Get the Dressing Ready:**
   - ❖ Combine Greek yogurt, olive oil, minced garlic, lemon juice, Dijon mustard, salt, and pepper in a small bowl.

2. **Assemble the Salad:**
   - ❖ Toss the romaine lettuce with the dressing in a big bowl until evenly coated.
   - ❖ Add whole wheat croutons and shaved Parmesan cheese over top.

3. **Provide:**
   - ❖ Present right away.

## Ingredient Alternatives and Substitutes:

I. **Legume Romaine:** Replace with kale or mixed greens.

II. **Parmesan Cheese:** To make a dairy-free variation, use nutritional yeast.

III. **Greek Yogurt:** Use sour cream or a dairy-free yogurt in its place.

## Nutritional Information:

- 180 calories
- 9g of protein
- 20g of carbohydrates
- 4g of dietary fiber
- 4g of sugars
- 8g of fat
- 2g of saturated fat
- 350 mg of sodium
- 300 milligrams of potassium
- 30% DV for vitamin A
- 20% DV for vitamin C
- Iron: 8% DV

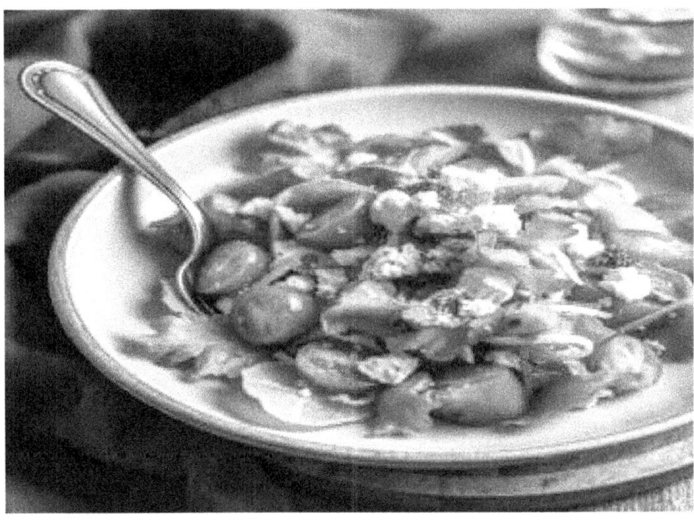

# Warm Lentil and Sweet Potato Salad

Serving: four

Prep Time: 30 minutes

Cooking Time: 15 minutes

## Ingredients:

- one cup of brown or green lentils, dry
- Two and a half cups of water
- One big sweet potato, chopped and skinned
- Two tsp olive oil
- Half a teaspoon of cumin powder
- One-half tsp paprika
- To taste, add salt and black pepper.
- 1/4 cup finely chopped fresh parsley
– Two tsp red wine vinegar

## How to Prepare:

### 1. Prepare the Lentils:
- ❖ Rinse the lentils under cold running water.
- ❖ Fill a medium pot with the lentils and water. After bringing to a boil, lower the heat, and simmer until the food is soft, 20 to 25 minutes. After draining, set away.

### 2. Sweetheart Potato Roast:
- ❖ Set oven temperature to 200°C/400°F.
- ❖ Combine olive oil, salt, pepper, cumin, and paprika with the sweet potato cubes.
- ❖ Spread out on a baking sheet and roast until soft, 25 to 30 minutes.

### 3. Assemble the Salad:
- ❖ Combine cooked lentils, roasted sweet potatoes, and parsley straight into a big bowl.
- ❖ Pour in some red wine vinegar and mix well.

### 4. Provide:
- ❖ You can serve it hot or at room temperature.

## Ingredient Alternatives and Substitutes:

I. **Lentils:** Use black beans or chickpeas in their place.
II. **Sweet Potato:** You can use ordinary potatoes or butternut squash.

## Nutritional Information:

- 250 calories
- 12g of protein
- 40g of carbohydrates
- 10g of dietary fiber
- 8g of sugars
- 8g of fat
- 1g of saturated fat
- 150 milligrams of sodium
- 600 mg of potassium
- 80% DV for vitamin A
- 30% DV for vitamin C
- Iron: 25% DV

# Roasted Brussels Sprouts with Balsamic Glaze

Serving: four

Prep Time: 25 minutes

Cooking Time: Ten minutes

## Ingredients:

- One pound of clipped and cut-in-half Brussels sprouts
- Two tsp olive oil
- To taste, add salt and black pepper.
- One-fourth cup of balsamic vinegar
- One tablespoon of honey

## How to Prepare:

### 1. Sprouts should be roasted:

- ❖ Set oven temperature to 200°C/400°F.
- ❖ Combine salt, pepper, and olive oil with the Brussels sprouts.
- ❖ Transfer to a baking sheet, then roast for 20 to 25 minutes, or until golden and crispy.

### 2. Get the Balsamic Glaze Ready:

- ❖ Combine honey and balsamic vinegar in a small pot.
- ❖ Reduce by half and cook for 5 to 7 minutes, or until syrupy, after bringing to a simmer.

### 3. Provide:

- ❖ Gently mix the roasted Brussels sprouts with a drizzle of the balsamic glaze.

## Ingredient Alternatives and Substitutes:

I. **Brussels sprouts:** Use cauliflower florets in place of sprouts.
II. **Balsamic Vinegar:** To add a distinct flavor, substitute red wine vinegar.

## Nutritional Information:

- 150 calories
- 4g of protein
- 20g of carbohydrates
- 6g of dietary fiber
- 12g of sugars
- 6g of fat
- 1g of saturated fat
- 200 milligrams of sodium
- 500 milligrams of potassium
- 10% DV for vitamin A
- Vitamin C: 80% of the DV
- Iron: 8% DV

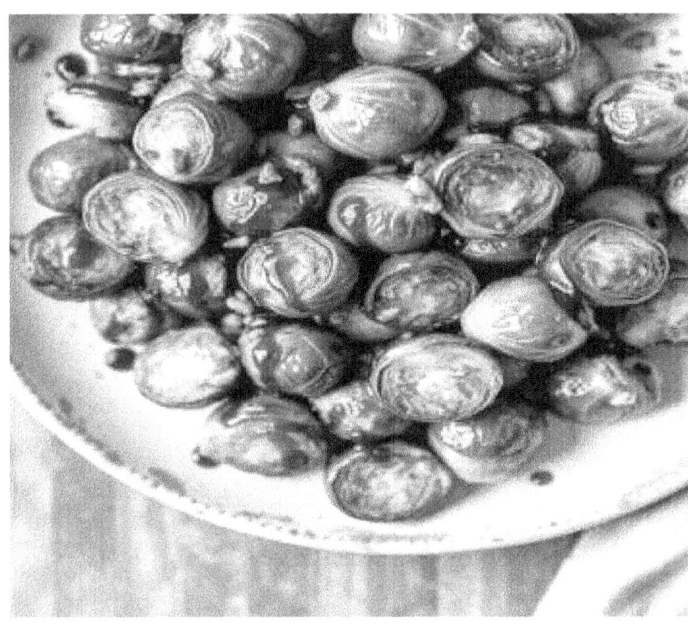

# Steamed Asparagus with Lemon

🍴 Serving: four

⏱ Prep Time: Five minutes

⏱ Cooking Time: Five minutes

## Ingredients:

- One trimmed bunch of asparagus

- One tablespoon of olive oil

- One lemon's juice

- To taste, add salt and black pepper.

## How to Prepare:

### 1. Cook the asparagus:

- ❖ Put the asparagus in a steamer basket and steam it over boiling water for four to five minutes, or until it is crisp-tender.

### 2. Attain and Present:

- ❖ Move the asparagus to a dish for serving.
- ❖ Pour olive oil and lemon juice over.
- ❖ Season to taste with salt and pepper.

## Ingredient Alternatives and Substitutes:

I. **Asparagus:** Swap for broccoli or green beans.

II. **Lemon Juice:** For a variation in flavor, substitute white wine vinegar.

## Nutritional Information:

- 60 calories
- 3g of protein
- 6g of carbohydrates
- 3g of dietary fiber
- 2g of sugars
- 3g of fat
- Saturated Fat: 0 g
- Sodium: 0 mg
- 300 milligrams of potassium
- 15% DV for vitamin A
- 20% DV for vitamin C
- Iron: 10% DV

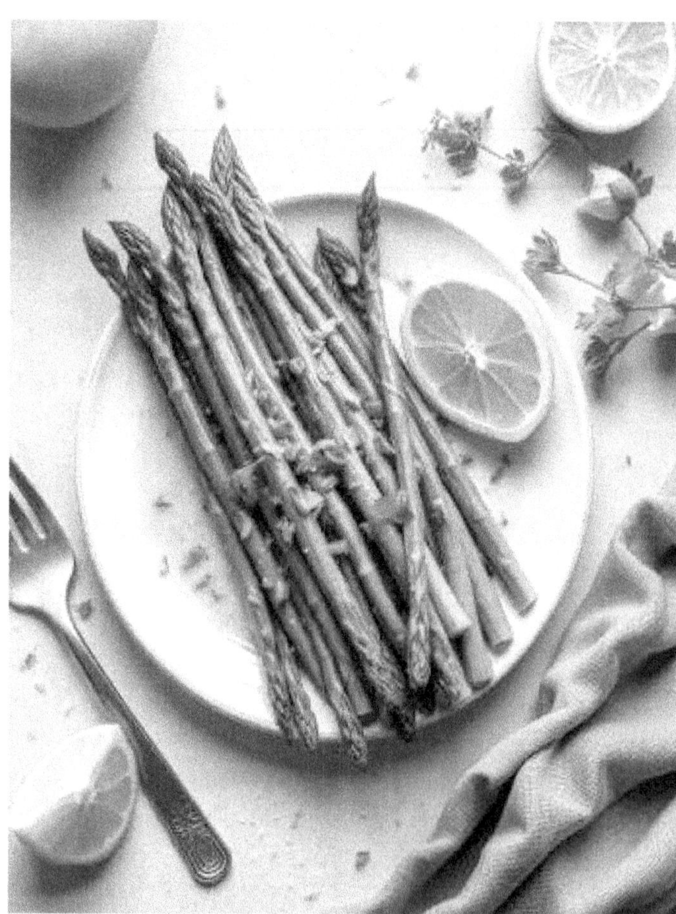

# Garlic and Herb Mashed Cauliflower

Serving: four

Prep Time: 15  minutes

Cooking Time: Ten minutes

## Ingredients:

- One large head of cauliflower, divided into pieces.
- Three minced garlic cloves
- Two tsp olive oil
- 1/4 cup of freshly chopped parsley
- To taste, add salt and black pepper.

## How to Prepare:

### 1. Get the cauliflower cooked:

- ❖ Pour the boiling water over the cauliflower florets in a big pot.
- ❖ Simmer for ten to twelve minutes, or until soft.

### 2. Season and Mash:

- ❖ After draining, add the cauliflower back to the saucepan.
- ❖ Add olive oil and minced garlic. Smoothly mash with an immersion blender or a potato masher.
- ❖ Add the pepper, salt, and chopped parsley and stir.

### 3. Provide:

- ❖ As an accompaniment, serve warm.

## Ingredient Alternatives and Substitutes:

I. **Carrot:** Instead of using a typical mash, use steaming potatoes.
II. **Olive Oil:** Use butter or a substitute that is free of dairy.

## Nutritional Information:

- 100 calories
- 3g of protein
- 10g of carbohydrates
- 4g of dietary fiber
- 3g of sugars
- 6g of fat
- 1g of saturated fat
- 200 milligrams of sodium
- 300 milligrams of potassium
- 10% DV for vitamin A
- Vitamin C: 80% of the DV
- Iron: 6% DV

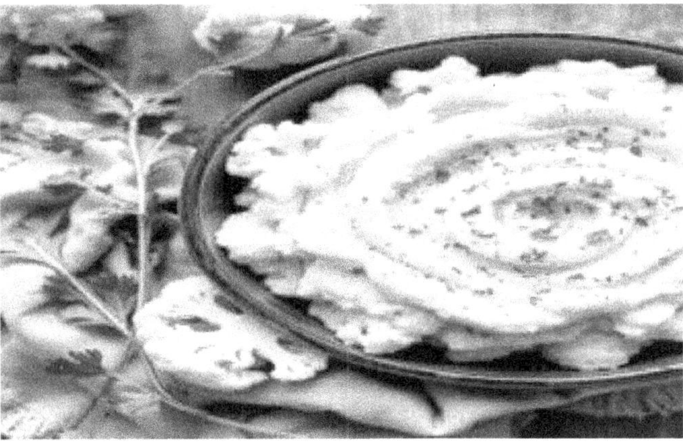

# Spicy Chickpea and Avocado Salad

Serving: four

Prep Time: N/B

Cooking Time: Ten minutes

## Ingredients:

- One 15-oz can of washed and drained chickpeas
- One diced avocado
- Half a red onion, diced finely
- Half a cup of cherry tomatoes
- One tablespoon of olive oil
- One tablespoon of lime juice
- One tsp of paprika with smoke
- Half a teaspoon of optional cayenne
- To taste, add salt and black pepper.
- To garnish, fresh cilantro

## How to Prepare:

### 1. Mix the Ingredients:

- ❖ Combine the avocado, cherry tomatoes, red onion, and chickpeas in a big bowl.

### 2. Get the Dressing Ready:

- ❖ Combine the olive oil, lime juice, smoked paprika, salt, pepper, and cayenne (if using) in a small bowl.

### 3. Discard and Present:

- ❖ Pour the dressing over the salad and toss lightly.
- ❖ Add some fresh cilantro as a garnish.

## Ingredient Alternatives and Substitutes:

I. **Chickpeas:** Use kidney or black beans as a substitute.
II. **Avocado:** To provide a distinct texture, substitute sliced cucumber.

## Nutritional Information:

- 220 calories
- 8g of protein
- 25g of carbohydrates
- 8g of dietary fiber
- 4g of sugars
- 10g of fat
- 1g of saturated fat
- 200 milligrams of sodium
- 400 milligrams of potassium
- 15% DV for vitamin A
- 20% DV for vitamin C
- Iron: 15% DV

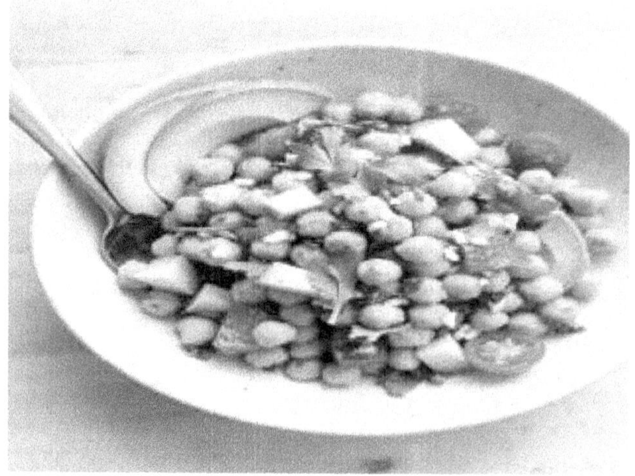

# Chapter 4: Soups and Stews

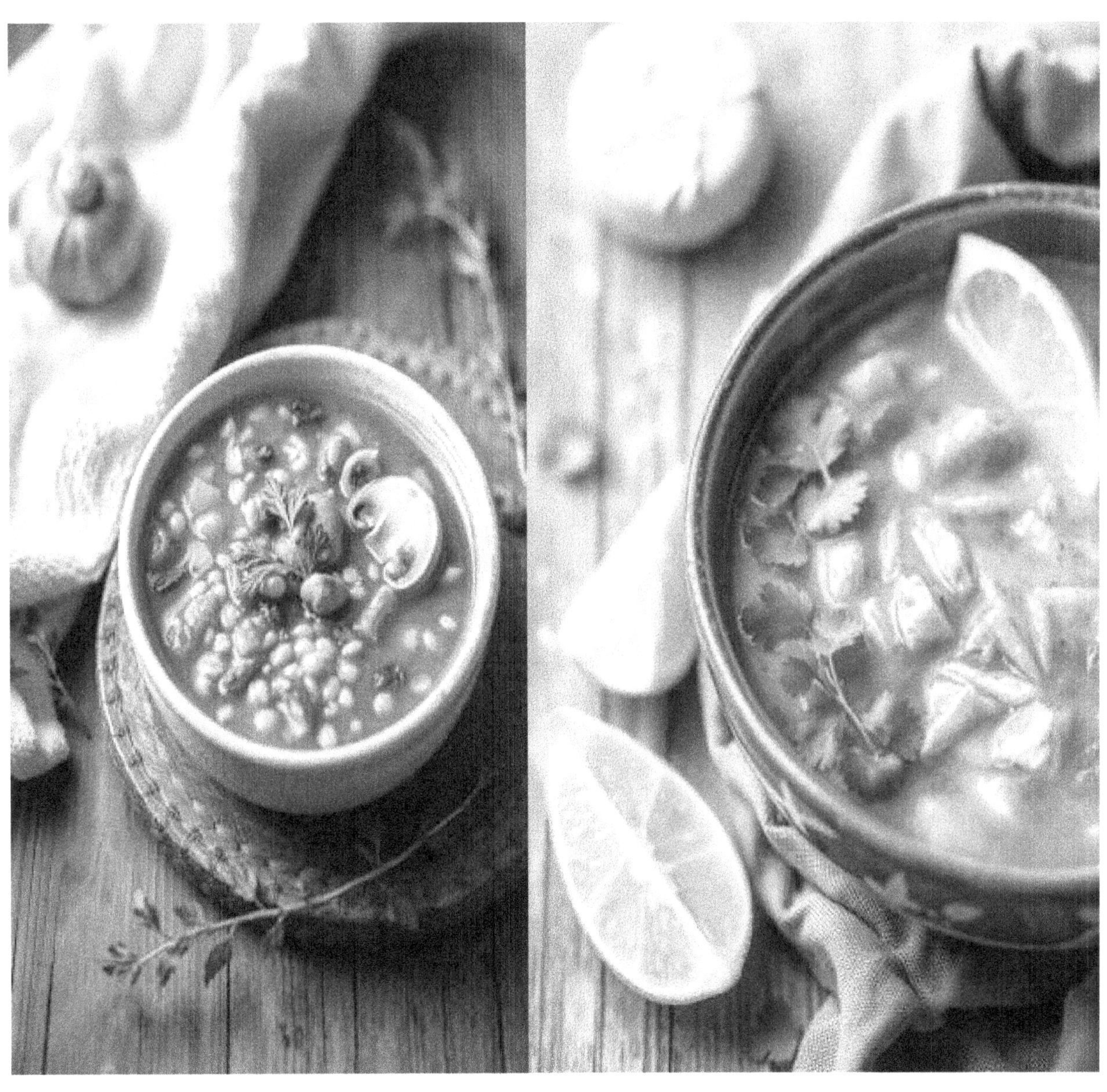

# Hearty Vegetable Soup

Serving: Six

Prep Time: 15 minutes

Cooking Time: 30 minutes

## Ingredients:

- 1 tablespoon olive oil
- 1 onion, diced
- 2 cloves garlic, minced
- 3 carrots, peeled and diced
- 2 celery stalks, diced
- 1 zucchini, diced
- 1 bell pepper, diced
- 1 cup green beans, chopped
- 1 cup diced tomatoes (canned or fresh)
- 6 cups vegetable broth
- 1 teaspoon dried thyme
- 1 teaspoon dried basil
- Salt and black pepper to taste
- 1 cup chopped fresh spinach

## How to Prepare:

1. **Sauté the Vegetables:**
   - ❖ In a large pot, heat olive oil over medium heat.
   - ❖ Add onion and garlic and sauté until softened, about 5 minutes.

2. **Cook the Soup:**
   - ❖ Add carrots, celery, zucchini, bell pepper, and green beans to the pot.
   - ❖ Sauté for an additional 5 minutes.
   - ❖ Stir in diced tomatoes, vegetable broth, thyme, basil, salt, and pepper.
   - ❖ Bring to a boil, then reduce heat and simmer for 20-25 minutes, or until vegetables are tender.

3. **Add Spinach:**
   - ❖ Stir in chopped spinach and cook for another 5 minutes, until wilted.

4. **Serve:**
   - ❖ Serve hot.

## Ingredients Substitutes and Alternatives:

I. **Vegetable Broth:** Use chicken broth for a different flavor.

II. **Spinach:** Substitute with kale or Swiss chard.

## Nutritional Information

- Calories: 120
- Protein: 4g
- Carbohydrates: 25g
- Dietary Fiber: 6g
- Sugars: 7g
- Fat: 3g
- Saturated Fat: 0.5g
- Sodium: 600mg
- Potassium: 600mg
- Vitamin A: 80% DV
- Vitamin C: 50% DV
- Iron: 10% DV

# Chicken and Wild Rice Soup

Serving: 6

Prep Time: 15  minutes

Cooking Time: 40 minutes

## Ingredients:

- 1 tablespoon olive oil
- 1 onion, diced
- 2 cloves garlic, minced
- 1 cup diced carrots
- 1 cup diced celery
- 1 cup wild rice
- 1 pound chicken breast, cooked and shredded
- 6 cups chicken broth
- 1 teaspoon dried thyme
- 1/2 teaspoon dried rosemary
- Salt and black pepper to taste
- 1 cup chopped fresh parsley

## How to Prepare:

1. **Sauté the Vegetables:**
   - ❖ In a large pot, heat olive oil over medium heat.
   - ❖ Add onion and garlic and sauté until softened, about 5 minutes.

2. **Cook the Soup:**
   - ❖ Add carrots and celery and cook for another 5 minutes.
   - ❖ Stir in wild rice, shredded chicken, chicken broth, thyme, rosemary, salt, and pepper.
   - ❖ Bring to a boil, then reduce heat and simmer for 30-35 minutes, or until rice is tender.

3. **Finish the Soup**:
   - ❖ Stir in fresh parsley and cook for another 5 minutes.

4. **Serve:**
   - ❖ Serve hot.

## Ingredients Substitutes and Alternatives:

I. **Wild Rice:** Substitute with brown rice or quinoa.

II. **Chicken Breast:** Use rotisserie chicken or leftover turkey.

## Nutritional Information;

- Calories: 250
- Protein: 20g
- Carbohydrates: 30g
- Dietary Fiber: 3g
- Sugars: 6g
- Fat: 8g
- Saturated Fat: 1g
- Sodium: 700mg
- Potassium: 600mg
- Vitamin A: 50% DV
- Vitamin C: 20% DV
- Iron: 15% DV

# Creamy Tomato Basil Soup

Serving: four

Prep Time: 10 minutes

Cooking Time: 25 minutes

## Ingredients:

- 1 tablespoon olive oil
- 1 onion, diced
- 3 cloves garlic, minced
- 2 cans (14.5 oz each) diced tomatoes
- 2 cups low-sodium vegetable broth
- 1 cup unsweetened almond milk (or whole milk)
- 1/4 cup fresh basil leaves, chopped
- 1/2 teaspoon dried oregano
- Salt and black pepper to taste

## How to Prepare:

### 1. Sauté the Aromatics:
- ❖ In a large pot, heat olive oil over medium heat.
- ❖ Add onion and garlic and cook until softened, about 5 minutes.

### 2. Cook the Soup:
- ❖ Stir in diced tomatoes, vegetable broth, and oregano. Bring to a boil.
- ❖ Reduce heat and simmer for 15 minutes.

### 3. Blend the Soup:
- ❖ Use an immersion blender to blend the soup until smooth (or blend in batches in a regular blender).

### 4. Add Creaminess:
- ❖ Stir in almond milk and cook for an additional 5 minutes.
- ❖ Add fresh basil and season with salt and pepper.

### 5. Serve:
- ❖ Serve hot with a drizzle of olive oil or a sprinkle of Parmesan cheese, if desired.

## Ingredients Substitutes and Alternatives:

I. **Almond Milk:** Use whole milk or coconut milk.

II. **Diced Tomatoes:** Substitute with crushed tomatoes for a smoother texture.

## Nutritional Information:

- Calories: 180
- Protein: 4g
- Carbohydrates: 20g
- Dietary Fiber: 4g
- Sugars: 10g
- Fat: 9g
- Saturated Fat: 1g
- Sodium: 500mg
- Potassium: 500mg
- Vitamin A: 30% DV
- Vitamin C: 50% DV
- Iron: 10% DV

# Lentil and Spinach Stew

Serving: four

Prep Time: 15 minutes

Cooking Time: 40 minutes

## Ingredients:

- 1 tablespoon olive oil
- 1 onion, diced
- 2 cloves garlic, minced
- 1 cup diced carrots
- 1 cup diced celery
- 1 cup dried green or brown lentils
- 6 cups vegetable broth
- 1 teaspoon ground cumin
- 1/2 teaspoon smoked paprika
- 2 cups fresh spinach, chopped
- Salt and black pepper to taste

## How to Prepare:

### 1. Sauté the Vegetables:

- ❖ In a large pot, heat olive oil over medium heat.
- ❖ Add onion and garlic and cook until softened, about 5 minutes.

### 2. Cook the Stew:

- ❖ Add carrots and celery and cook for another 5 minutes.
- ❖ Stir in lentils, vegetable broth, cumin, and paprika. Bring to a boil.
- ❖ Reduce heat and simmer for 30-35 minutes, or until lentils are tender.

### 3. Add Spinach:

- ❖ Stir in fresh spinach and cook for an additional 5 minutes until wilted.

### 4. Serve:

- ❖ Serve hot.

## Ingredients Substitutes and Alternatives:

I.  **Lentils:** Use chickpeas or black beans.
II. **Spinach:** Substitute with kale or Swiss chard.

## Nutritional Information (per serving):

- Calories: 220
- Protein: 12g
- Carbohydrates: 35g
- Dietary Fiber: 10g
- Sugars: 8g
- Fat: 6g
- Saturated Fat: 1g
- Sodium: 600mg
- Potassium: 700mg
- Vitamin A: 40% DV
- Vitamin C: 30% DV
- Iron: 25% DV

# Butternut Squash Soup

Serving: four

Prep Time: 15 minutes

Cooking Time: 30 minutes

## Ingredients:

- 1 tablespoon olive oil
- 1 onion, diced
- 2 cloves garlic, minced
- 1 large butternut squash, peeled, seeded, and cubed
- 4 cups vegetable broth
- 1/2 teaspoon ground nutmeg
- 1/2 teaspoon ground cinnamon
- Salt and black pepper to taste
- 1/2 cup unsweetened almond milk (or whole milk)

## How to Prepare:

### 1. Sauté the Aromatics:
- ❖ In a large pot, heat olive oil over medium heat.
- ❖ Add onion and garlic and cook until softened, about 5 minutes.

### 2. Cook the Squash:
- ❖ Add butternut squash and vegetable broth. Bring to a boil.
- ❖ Reduce heat and simmer for 20-25 minutes, or until squash is tender.

### 3. Blend the Soup:
- ❖ Use an immersion blender to blend the soup until smooth (or blend in batches in a regular blender).

### 4. Add Creaminess:
- ❖ Stir in almond milk, nutmeg, cinnamon, salt, and pepper. Cook for another 5 minutes.

### 5. Serve:
- ❖ Serve hot with a sprinkle of cinnamon or a drizzle of olive oil, if desired.

## Ingredients Substitutes and Alternatives:

I. **Butternut Squash:** Use pumpkin or sweet potatoes.

II. **Almond Milk:** Use coconut milk or whole milk.

## Nutritional Information :

- Calories: 180
- Protein: 3g
- Carbohydrates: 30g
- Dietary Fiber: 5g
- Sugars: 10g
- Fat: 7g
- Saturated Fat: 1g
- Sodium: 600mg
- Potassium: 600mg
- Vitamin A: 150% DV
- Vitamin C: 30% DV
- Iron: 10% DV

# Beef and Barley Stew

Serving: Six

Prep Time: 15  minutes

Cooking Time: 55 minutes

## Ingredients:

- 1 tablespoon olive oil
- 1 pound beef stew meat, cut into cubes
- 1 onion, diced
- 2 cloves garlic, minced
- 3 carrots, peeled and sliced
- 2 celery stalks, sliced
- 1 cup barley
- 6 cups beef broth
- 1 teaspoon dried thyme
- 1 teaspoon dried rosemary
- Salt and black pepper to taste
- 1 cup frozen peas

## How to Prepare:

### 1. Brown the Beef:
- ❖ In a large pot, heat olive oil over medium heat.
- ❖ Add beef and brown on all sides, about 5 minutes.

### 2. Cook the Stew:
- ❖ Add onion and garlic and cook until softened, about 5 minutes.
- ❖ Stir in carrots, celery, barley, beef broth, thyme, rosemary, salt, and pepper.
- ❖ Bring to a boil, then reduce heat and simmer for 45-50 minutes, or until beef and barley are tender.

### 3. Add Peas:
- ❖ Stir in frozen peas and cook for an additional 5 minutes.

### 4. Serve:
- ❖ Serve hot.

## Ingredients Substitutes and Alternatives:

I. **Beef Stew Meat:** Use chicken breast or tofu for a lighter option.

II. **Barley:** Substitute with brown rice or quinoa.

## Nutritional Information :

- Calories: 320
- Protein: 25g
- Carbohydrates: 30g
- Dietary Fiber: 8g
- Sugars: 6g
- Fat: 12g
- Saturated Fat: 4g
- Sodium: 800mg
- Potassium: 700mg
- Vitamin A: 60% DV
- Vitamin C: 20% DV
- Iron: 20% DV

# Spicy Black Bean Soup

Serving: four

Prep Time: 10 minutes

Cooking Time: 25 minutes

## Ingredients:

- 1 tablespoon olive oil
- 1 onion, diced
- 2 cloves garlic, minced
- 1 bell pepper, diced
- 1 can (15 oz) black beans, drained and rinsed
- 1 can (14.5 oz) diced tomatoes
- 4 cups vegetable broth
- 1 teaspoon ground cumin
- 1/2 teaspoon chili powder
- 1/4 teaspoon cayenne pepper (optional)
- Salt and black pepper to taste
- 1/4 cup chopped fresh cilantro

## How to Prepare:

### 1. Sauté the Aromatics:

❖ In a large pot, heat olive oil over medium heat.
❖ Add onion and garlic and cook until softened, about 5 minutes.

### 2. Cook the Soup:

❖ Add bell pepper and cook for another 5 minutes.
❖ Stir in black beans, diced tomatoes, vegetable broth, cumin, chili powder, cayenne pepper (if using), salt, and pepper.
❖ Bring to a boil, then reduce heat and simmer for 20-25 minutes.

### 3. Finish the Soup:

❖ Stir in fresh cilantro.

### 4. Serve:

❖ Serve hot.

## Ingredients Substitutes and Alternatives:

I. **Black Beans:** Substitute with kidney beans or chickpeas.
II. **Bell Pepper:** Use diced carrots or celery.

## Nutritional Information :

- Calories: 220
- Protein: 12g
- Carbohydrates: 30g
- Dietary Fiber: 8g
- Sugars: 6g
- Fat: 6g
- Saturated Fat: 1g
- Sodium: 500mg
- Potassium: 700mg
- Vitamin A: 20% DV
- Vitamin C: 40% DV
- Iron: 15% DV

# Mushroom and Barley Soup

Serving: four

Prep Time: 10 minutes

Cooking Time: 40 minutes

## Ingredients:

- 1 tablespoon olive oil
- 1 onion, diced
- 2 cloves garlic, minced
- 8 ounces mushrooms, sliced
- 1 cup barley
- 4 cups vegetable broth
- 1 cup water
- 1/2 teaspoon dried thyme
- Salt and black pepper to taste
- 1 cup chopped fresh parsley

## How to Prepare:

### 1. Sauté the Aromatics:

- ❖ In a large pot, heat olive oil over medium heat.
- ❖ Add onion and garlic and cook until softened, about 5 minutes.

### 2. Cook the Mushrooms:

- ❖ Add mushrooms and cook until tender, about 5 minutes.

### 3. Cook the Soup:

- ❖ Stir in barley, vegetable broth, water, thyme, salt, and pepper.
- ❖ Bring to a boil, then reduce heat and simmer for 30-35 minutes, or until barley is tender.

### 4. Finish the Soup:

- ❖ Stir in fresh parsley.

### 5. Serve:

- ❖ Serve hot.

## Ingredients Substitutes and Alternatives:

I. **Barley:** Substitute with brown rice or quinoa.

II. **Mushrooms:** Use diced tofu or extra vegetables.

## Nutritional Information:

- Calories: 220
- Protein: 8g
- Carbohydrates: 30g
- Dietary Fiber: 6g
- Sugars: 5g
- Fat: 6g
- Saturated Fat: 1g
- Sodium: 400mg
- Potassium: 500mg
- Vitamin A: 15% DV
- Vitamin C: 20% DV
- Iron: 12% DV

# Minestrone Soup

Serving: 6

Prep Time: 15  minutes

Cooking Time: 30 minutes

## Ingredients:

- 1 tablespoon olive oil
- 1 onion, diced
- 2 cloves garlic, minced
- 1 cup diced carrots
- 1 cup diced celery
- 1 cup green beans, chopped
- 1 can (14.5 oz) diced tomatoes
- 4 cups vegetable broth
- 1 cup cooked pasta (whole wheat or gluten-free)
- 1 can (15 oz) kidney beans, drained and rinsed
- 1/2 teaspoon dried oregano
- 1/2 teaspoon dried basil
- Salt and black pepper to taste
- 1 cup chopped fresh spinach

## How to Prepare:

### 1. Sauté the Vegetables:

❖ In a large pot, heat olive oil over medium heat.

❖ Add onion and garlic and cook until softened, about 5 minutes.

### 2. Cook the Soup:

❖ Add carrots, celery, and green beans and cook for another 5 minutes.

❖ Stir in diced tomatoes, vegetable broth, and oregano.

❖ Bring to a boil, then reduce heat and simmer for 20-25 minutes.

### 3. Add Pasta and Beans:

❖ Stir in cooked pasta, kidney beans, and spinach. Cook for another 5 minutes until heated through.

### 4. Serve:

❖ Serve hot.

## Ingredients Substitutes and Alternatives:

I. **Pasta:** Use quinoa or rice for a gluten-free option.

II. **Kidney Beans:** Substitute with chickpeas or black beans.

## Nutritional Information :

- Calories: 250
- Protein: 12g
- Carbohydrates: 40g
- Dietary Fiber: 8g
- Sugars: 10g
- Fat: 6g
- Saturated Fat: 1g
- Sodium: 600mg
- Potassium: 700mg
- Vitamin A: 50% DV
- Vitamin C: 25% DV
- Iron: 15% DV

# Chicken Tortilla Soup

Serving: 6

Prep Time: 15 minutes

Cooking Time: 25 minutes

## Ingredients:

- 1 tablespoon olive oil
- 1 onion, diced
- 2 cloves garlic, minced
- 1 bell pepper, diced
- 1 can (15 oz) diced tomatoes
- 4 cups chicken broth
- 1 cup shredded cooked chicken
- 1 cup corn kernels (fresh or frozen)
- 1/2 teaspoon ground cumin
- 1/2 teaspoon chili powder
- Salt and black pepper to taste
- 1/4 cup chopped fresh cilantro
- 1 cup tortilla chips, crushed (for serving)
- Lime wedges (for garnish)

## How to Prepare:

1. **Sauté the Aromatics:**
   - ❖ In a large pot, heat olive oil over medium heat.
   - ❖ Add onion and garlic and cook until softened, about 5 minutes.

2. **Cook the Soup:**
   - ❖ Add bell pepper and cook for another 5 minutes.
   - ❖ Stir in diced tomatoes, chicken broth, shredded chicken, corn, cumin, and chili powder.
   - ❖ Bring to a boil, then reduce heat and simmer for 20 minutes.

3. **Finish the Soup:**
   - ❖ Stir in fresh cilantro.

4. Serve:
   - ❖ Ladle soup into bowls and top with crushed tortilla chips and lime wedges.

## Ingredients Substitutes and Alternatives:

I. **Chicken Broth:** Use vegetable broth for a vegetarian version.

II. **Tortilla Chips:** Use whole-grain crackers or omit for a lower-calorie option.

## Nutritional Information :

- Calories: 290
- Protein: 20g
- Carbohydrates: 30g
- Dietary Fiber: 6g
- Sugars: 8g
- Fat: 10g
- Saturated Fat: 1.5g
- Sodium: 700mg
- Potassium: 600mg
- Vitamin A: 40% DV
- Vitamin C: 25% DV
- Iron: 15% DV

# Chapter 5: Main Dishes

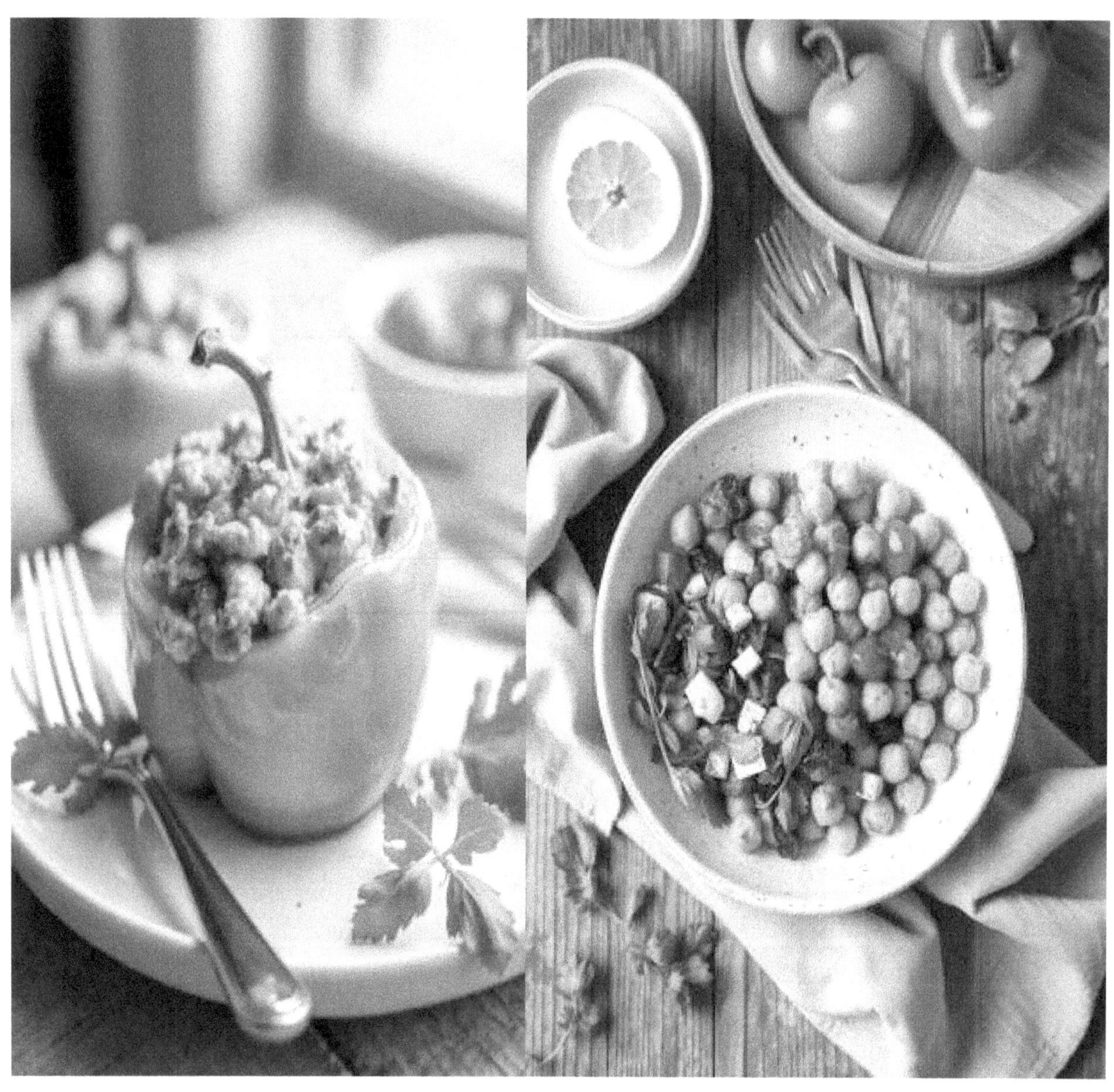

# Grilled Lemon Herb Chicken

Serving: 4

Prep Time: 10 minutes

Cooking Time: 15 minutes

## Ingredients:

- 4 boneless, skinless chicken breasts
- 1/4 cup olive oil
- Juice of 2 lemons
- 3 cloves garlic, minced
- 1 tablespoon dried oregano
- 1 tablespoon dried rosemary
- 1 teaspoon dried thyme
- Salt and black pepper to taste

## How to Prepare:

### 1. Marinate the Chicken:

- ❖ In a bowl, combine olive oil, lemon juice, garlic, oregano, rosemary, thyme, salt, and pepper.
- ❖ Place chicken breasts in a resealable plastic bag or shallow dish and pour marinade over them.
- ❖ Seal the bag or cover the dish and refrigerate for at least 1 hour, preferably overnight.

### 2. Grill the Chicken:

- ❖ Preheat the grill to medium-high heat.
- ❖ Remove chicken from marinade and discard excess marinade.
- ❖ Grill chicken for 6-7 minutes per side, or until the internal temperature reaches 165°F (75°C).

### 3. Serve:

- ❖ Serve hot, garnished with additional lemon wedges and fresh herbs if desired.

## Ingredients Substitutes and Alternatives:

I. **Olive Oil:** Use avocado oil or canola oil.

II. **Chicken Breasts**: Substitute with thighs or a plant-based protein.

## Nutritional Information:

- Calories: 230
- Protein: 30g
- Carbohydrates: 2g
- Dietary Fiber: 0g
- Sugars: 0g
- Fat: 12g
- Saturated Fat: 2g
- Sodium: 150mg
- Potassium: 350mg
- Vitamin C: 15% DV
- Iron: 6% DV

# Baked Salmon with Dill

🍴 Serving: four

⏱ Prep Time: 10 minutes

⏱ Cooking Time: 20 minutes

## Ingredients:

- 4 salmon fillets
- 2 tablespoons olive oil
- Juice of 1 lemon
- 2 cloves garlic, minced
- 2 tablespoons fresh dill, chopped (or 1 tablespoon dried dill)
- Salt and black pepper to taste

## How to Prepare:

1. **Preheat Oven:**
   - ❖ Preheat the oven to 375°F (190°C).

2. **Prepare the Salmon:**
   - ❖ Place salmon fillets on a baking sheet lined with parchment paper.
   - ❖ In a small bowl, mix olive oil, lemon juice, garlic, dill, salt, and pepper.
   - ❖ Brush the mixture over the salmon fillets.

3. **Bake the Salmon:**
   - ❖ Bake for 15-20 minutes, or until the salmon flakes easily with a fork and reaches an internal temperature of 145°F (63°C).

4. **Serve:**
   - ❖ Serve hot, garnished with additional dill and lemon wedges if desired.

## Ingredients Substitutes and Alternatives:

I. **Salmon:** Substitute with trout or another firm fish.
II. **Dill:** Use fresh parsley or thyme if dill is unavailable.

## Nutritional Information:

- Calories: 280
- Protein: 25g
- Carbohydrates: 2g
- Dietary Fiber: 0g
- Sugars: 0g
- Fat: 20g
- Saturated Fat: 3g
- Sodium: 80mg
- Potassium: 500mg
- Vitamin D: 50% DV
- Omega-3: 1.5g

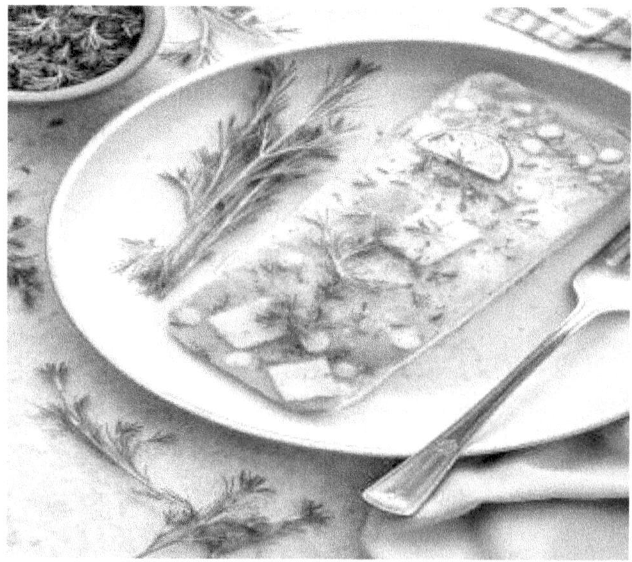

# Stuffed Bell Peppers

Serving: four

Prep Time: 15 minutes

Cooking Time: 40 minutes

## Ingredients:

- 4 large bell peppers (any color)
- 1 tablespoon olive oil
- 1 onion, diced
- 2 cloves garlic, minced
- 1 cup cooked brown rice
- 1 can (15 oz) black beans, drained and rinsed
- 1 cup corn kernels (fresh or frozen)
- 1 cup diced tomatoes
- 1 teaspoon ground cumin
- 1/2 teaspoon chili powder
- Salt and black pepper to taste
- 1/2 cup shredded low-fat cheese (optional)

## How to Prepare:

1. **Preheat Oven:**
   - ❖ Preheat the oven to 375°F (190°C).

2. **Prepare the Peppers:**
   - ❖ Cut the tops off the bell peppers and remove seeds and membranes.
   - ❖ Place the peppers cut side up in a baking dish.

3. **Prepare the Filling:**
   - ❖ In a large skillet, heat olive oil over medium heat.
   - ❖ Add onion and garlic and cook until softened, about 5 minutes.
   - ❖ Stir in cooked rice, black beans, corn, tomatoes, cumin, chili powder, salt, and pepper. Cook for an additional 5 minutes.

4. **Stuff the Peppers:**
   - ❖ Spoon the filling into each bell pepper. Sprinkle with shredded cheese if using.

5. **Bake the Peppers:**
   - ❖ Cover with foil and bake for 30 minutes.
   - ❖ Remove foil and bake for an additional 10 minutes, or until peppers are tender and cheese is melted.

6. **Serve:**
   - ❖ Serve hot.

## Ingredients Substitutes and Alternatives:

I. **Brown Rice:** Substitute with quinoa or couscous.

II. **Black Beans:** Use kidney beans or chickpeas.

III. **Cheese:** Omit for a dairy-free version or use a vegan cheese alternative

## Nutritional Information

- Calories: 250
- Protein: 10g
- Carbohydrates: 40g
- Dietary Fiber: 8g
- Sugars: 7g
- Fat: 7g
- Saturated Fat: 1g
- Sodium: 300mg
- Potassium: 600mg
- Vitamin A: 100% DV
- Vitamin C: 150% DV
- Iron: 15% DV

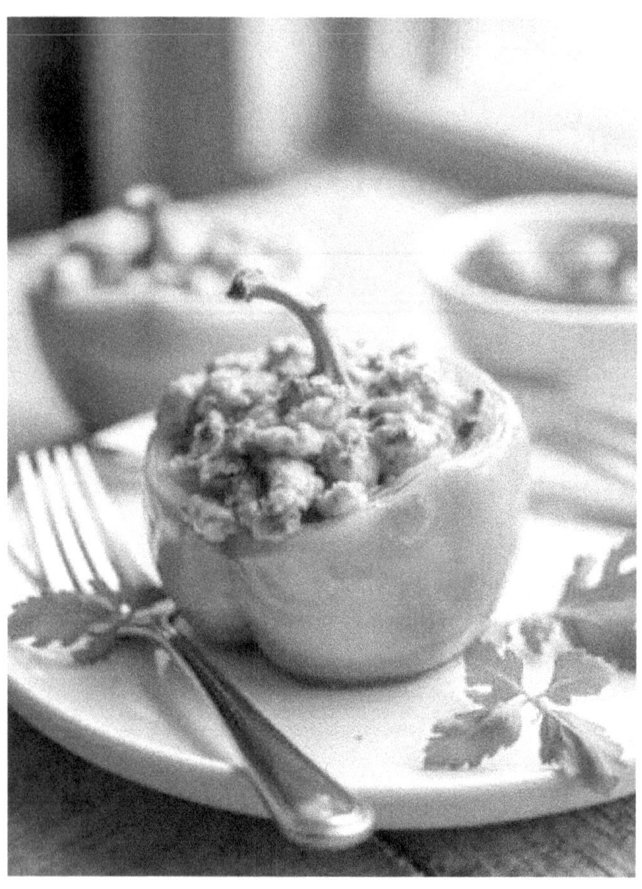

# Mediterranean Chickpea Bowl

Serving: four

Prep Time: 10 minutes

Cooking Time: 25 minutes

## Ingredients:

- 1 can (15 oz) chickpeas, drained and rinsed
- 1 tablespoon olive oil
- 1 teaspoon ground cumin
- 1/2 teaspoon smoked paprika
- Salt and black pepper to taste
- 1 cup cooked quinoa
- 1/2 cup diced cucumber
- 1/2 cup cherry tomatoes, halved
- 1/4 cup Kalamata olives, sliced
- 1/4 cup crumbled feta cheese (optional)
- 2 tablespoons chopped fresh parsley
- Lemon wedges for serving

## How to Prepare:

1. **Prepare the Chickpeas:**
   - ❖ Preheat the oven to 400°F (200°C).
   - ❖ In a bowl, toss chickpeas with olive oil, cumin, paprika, salt, and pepper.
   - ❖ Spread on a baking sheet and roast for 20-25 minutes, or until crispy.

2. **Assemble the Bowl:**
   - ❖ In a bowl, layer quinoa, roasted chickpeas, cucumber, cherry tomatoes, olives, and feta cheese if using.

3. **Garnish:**

❖ Sprinkle with chopped parsley and serve with lemon wedges.

## Ingredients Substitutes and Alternatives:

I. **Chickpeas:** Substitute with lentils or black beans.
II. **Quinoa:** Use brown rice or couscous.
III. **Feta Cheese:** Omit for a dairy-free version or use vegan feta.

## Nutritional Information :

- Calories: 350
- Protein: 12g
- Carbohydrates: 45g
- Dietary Fiber: 10g
- Sugars: 6g
- Fat: 12g
- Saturated Fat: 2g
- Sodium: 400mg
- Potassium: 600mg
- Vitamin C: 40% DV
- Vitamin A: 15% DV
- Iron: 20% DV

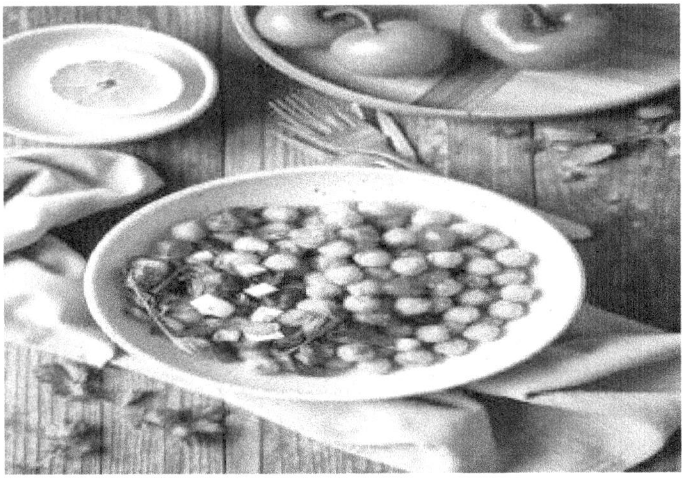

# Turkey and Spinach Meatballs

Serving: four

Prep Time: 10 minutes

Cooking Time: 25 minutes

## Ingredients:

- 1 pound ground turkey
- 1 cup fresh spinach, finely chopped
- 1/2 cup whole wheat breadcrumbs
- 1/4 cup grated Parmesan cheese (optional)
- 1 egg, beaten
- 2 cloves garlic, minced
- 1 teaspoon dried oregano
- Salt and black pepper to taste
- 1 tablespoon olive oil (for cooking)

## How to Prepare:

1. **Preheat Oven:**
   ❖ Preheat the oven to 375°F (190°C).

2. **Prepare the Meatballs:**
   ❖ In a large bowl, combine ground turkey, spinach, breadcrumbs, Parmesan cheese, egg, garlic, oregano, salt, and pepper.
   ❖ Mix until well combined.

3. **Form and Bake:**
   ❖ Shape mixture into 1-inch meatballs and place on a baking sheet.
   ❖ Bake for 20-25 minutes, or until meatballs are cooked through and have an internal temperature of 165°F (75°C).

## 4. Serve:

- ❖ Serve hot with marinara sauce or as desired.

## Ingredients Substitutes and Alternatives:

I. **Ground Turkey:** Use ground chicken or lean beef.
II. **Whole Wheat Breadcrumbs:** Use gluten-free breadcrumbs or crushed oats.

## Nutritional Information (per serving):

- Calories: 250
- Protein: 30g
- Carbohydrates: 10g
- Dietary Fiber: 2g
- Sugars: 1g
- Fat: 10g
- Saturated Fat: 3g
- Sodium: 200mg
- Potassium: 500mg
- Vitamin A: 20% DV
- Calcium: 15% DV
- Iron: 15% DV

# Eggplant Parmesan

Serving: four

Prep Time: 15 minutes

Cooking Time: 45 minutes

## Ingredients:

- 2 large eggplants, sliced into 1/2-inch rounds
- 1 cup whole wheat breadcrumbs
- 1/2 cup grated Parmesan cheese (optional)
- 2 cups marinara sauce
- 1 cup shredded part-skim mozzarella cheese
- 2 tablespoons olive oil
- 1 teaspoon dried basil
- 1 teaspoon dried oregano
- Salt and black pepper to taste

## How to Prepare:

### 1. Preheat Oven:

- ❖ Preheat the oven to 375°F (190°C).

### 2. Prepare Eggplant:

- ❖ Sprinkle eggplant slices with salt and let sit for 15 minutes to draw out moisture. Rinse and pat dry.
- ❖ Brush eggplant slices with olive oil and coat with breadcrumbs mixed with Parmesan cheese, basil, oregano, salt, and pepper.

3. **Bake the Eggplant:**
   - ❖ Place coated eggplant slices on a baking sheet and bake for 20 minutes, flipping halfway through.

4. **Assemble and Bake:**
   - ❖ In a baking dish, layer baked eggplant slices with marinara sauce and mozzarella cheese.
   - ❖ Bake for an additional 20-25 minutes, or until cheese is bubbly and golden.

5. **Serve:**
   - ❖ Serve hot with a side salad or whole grain pasta.

## Ingredients Substitutes and Alternatives:

I. **Eggplant:** Substitute with zucchini or portobello mushrooms.

II. **Whole Wheat Breadcrumbs:** Use gluten-free breadcrumbs or panko.

## Nutritional Information:

- Calories: 300
- Protein: 18g
- Carbohydrates: 30g
- Dietary Fiber: 8g
- Sugars: 8g
- Fat: 12g
- Saturated Fat: 5g
- Sodium: 700mg
- Potassium: 800mg
- Vitamin A: 15% DV
- Vitamin C: 30% DV
- Iron: 10% DV

# Grilled Shrimp Skewers

Serving: four

Prep Time: 15 minutes

Cooking Time: 6 minutes

## Ingredients:

- 1 pound large shrimp, peeled and deveined
- 2 tablespoons olive oil
- Juice of 1 lime
- 2 cloves garlic, minced
- 1 teaspoon smoked paprika
- 1/2 teaspoon ground cumin
- Salt and black pepper to taste
- Fresh cilantro for garnish

## How to Prepare:

1. **Marinate the Shrimp:**
   - ❖ In a bowl, combine olive oil, lime juice, garlic, paprika, cumin, salt, and pepper.
   - ❖ Add shrimp and toss to coat. Marinate for 15-30 minutes.

2. **Prepare the Skewers:**
   - ❖ Preheat the grill to medium-high heat.
   - ❖ Thread shrimp onto skewers.

3. **Grill the Shrimp:**
   - ❖ Grill shrimp for 2-3 minutes per side, or until they turn pink and opaque.

4. **Serve:**
  - ❖ Garnish with fresh cilantro and serve with a side of rice or a fresh salad.

## Ingredients Substitutes and Alternatives:

I. **Shrimp:** Substitute with chicken breast or tofu.
II. **Olive Oil:** Use avocado oil or canola oil.

## Nutritional Information:

- Calories: 180
- Protein: 25g
- Carbohydrates: 2g
- Dietary Fiber: 0g
- Sugars: 1g
- Fat: 8g
- Saturated Fat: 1g
- Sodium: 300mg
- Potassium: 300mg
- Vitamin C: 20% DV
- Iron: 10% DV

# Quinoa Stuffed Acorn Squash

Serving: four

Prep Time: 15 minutes

Cooking Time: 50 minutes

## Ingredients:

- 2 acorn squashes, halved and seeded
- 1 cup cooked quinoa
- 1/2 cup dried cranberries
- 1/4 cup chopped pecans
- 1/4 cup crumbled feta cheese (optional)
- 1 tablespoon olive oil
- 1/2 teaspoon ground cinnamon
- Salt and black pepper to taste

## How to Prepare:

1. **Preheat Oven:**
  - ❖ Preheat the oven to 400°F (200°C).

2. **Prepare the Squash:**
  - ❖ Brush the inside of the squash halves with olive oil and season with salt and pepper.
  - ❖ Place squash cut side down on a baking sheet and roast for 30-40 minutes, or until tender.

3. **Prepare the Filling:**
  - ❖ In a bowl, mix cooked quinoa, cranberries, pecans, and feta cheese if using.

4. **Stuff the Squash:**
   - ❖ Turn squash halves cut side up and fill with quinoa mixture.
   - ❖ Return to the oven and bake for an additional 10 minutes.

5. **Serve:**
   - ❖ Serve warm.

## Ingredients Substitutes and Alternatives:

I. **Quinoa:** Use cooked brown rice or couscous.

II. **Cranberries:** Substitute with raisins or chopped dates.

III. **Pecans:** Use walnuts or almonds.

## Nutritional Information:

- Calories: 300
- Protein: 10g
- Carbohydrates: 45g
- Dietary Fiber: 7g
- Sugars: 15g
- Fat: 10g
- Saturated Fat: 2g
- Sodium: 200mg
- Potassium: 600mg
- Vitamin A: 150% DV
- Vitamin C: 30% DV
- Iron: 15% DV

# Spicy Tofu Stir-Fry

Serving: four

Prep Time: 10 minutes

Cooking Time: 15 minutes

## Ingredients:

- 1 block (14 oz) firm tofu, cubed
- 2 tablespoons olive oil
- 1 red bell pepper, sliced
- 1 yellow bell pepper, sliced
- 1 cup broccoli florets
- 1 carrot, sliced
- 2 cloves garlic, minced
- 1 tablespoon soy sauce (low sodium)
- 1 tablespoon sriracha sauce (or to taste)
- 1 teaspoon ground ginger
- 2 green onions, sliced
- 1 tablespoon sesame seeds (optional)

## How to Prepare:

1. **Prepare the Tofu:**
   - ❖ In a large skillet or wok, heat olive oil over medium-high heat.
   - ❖ Add cubed tofu and cook until golden brown on all sides, about 5-7 minutes. Remove tofu and set aside.

2. **Cook the Vegetables:**
   - ❖ In the same skillet, add bell peppers, broccoli, carrot, and garlic. Stir-fry for 5 minutes, or until vegetables are tender-crisp.

3. **Add Tofu and Sauce:**
   - ❖ Return tofu to the skillet and stir in soy sauce, sriracha, and ground ginger.
   - ❖ Cook for an additional 2-3 minutes, until everything is heated through.

4. **Serve:**
   - ❖ Garnish with green onions and sesame seeds if using. Serve with brown rice or quinoa.

## Ingredients Substitutes and Alternatives:

I. **Tofu:** Substitute with tempeh or chicken breast.

II. **Sriracha:** Use hot sauce or chili flakes for a different heat level.

III. **Soy Sauce:** Use tamari or coconut aminos for a gluten-free option

## Nutritional Information:

- Calories: 250
- Protein: 15g
- Carbohydrates: 20g
- Dietary Fiber: 6g
- Sugars: 8g
- Fat: 15g
- Saturated Fat: 2g
- Sodium: 600mg
- Potassium: 600mg
- Vitamin A: 80% DV
- Vitamin C: 100% DV
- Iron: 15% DV

# Moroccan Lamb Tagine

Serving: four

Prep Time: 15 minutes

Cooking Time: 1 hour 15 minutes

## Ingredients:

- 1 pound lamb stew meat, cut into cubes
- 1 tablespoon olive oil
- 1 onion, diced
- 2 cloves garlic, minced
- 2 teaspoons ground cumin
- 1 teaspoon ground coriander
- 1 teaspoon ground cinnamon
- 1/2 teaspoon turmeric
- 1/2 teaspoon paprika
- 1/2 teaspoon black pepper
- 1 cup chopped tomatoes
- 1 cup chicken or vegetable broth
- 1/2 cup dried apricots, chopped
- 1/2 cup almonds, toasted
- 1 cup cooked couscous or quinoa

## How to Prepare:

1. **Brown the Lamb:**
   - ❖ Heat olive oil in a large pot or Dutch oven over medium heat.
   - ❖ Add lamb and cook until browned on all sides, about 8 minutes. Remove lamb and set aside.

2. **Cook the Aromatics:**
   - ❖ In the same pot, add onion and garlic. Cook until softened, about 5 minutes.

3. **Add Spices and Tomatoes:**
   - ❖ Stir in cumin, coriander, cinnamon, turmeric, paprika, and pepper.
   - ❖ Add chopped tomatoes and cook for 2 minutes.

4. **Simmer the Tagine:**
   - ❖ Return lamb to the pot. Add broth and dried apricots.
   - ❖ Bring to a boil, then reduce heat and simmer for 1 hour, or until lamb is tender.

5. **Finish and Serve:**
   - ❖ Stir in toasted almonds and serve over couscous or quinoa.

## Ingredients Substitutes and Alternatives:

I. **Lamb:** Substitute with beef or chicken.

II. **Dried Apricots:** Use raisins or dried dates.

III. **Couscous:** Use quinoa or brown rice.

## Nutritional Information :

- Calories: 350
- Protein: 25g
- Carbohydrates: 30g
- Dietary Fiber: 6g
- Sugars: 12g
- Fat: 15g
- Saturated Fat: 5g
- Sodium: 400mg
- Potassium: 600mg
- Vitamin A: 20% DV
- Vitamin C: 20% DV
- Iron: 25% DV

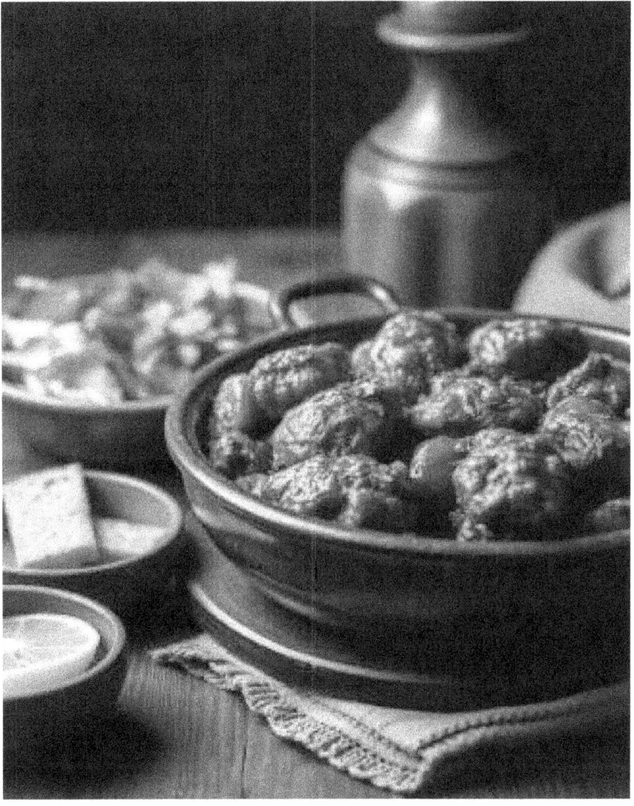

# Chapter 6: Snacks and Appetizers

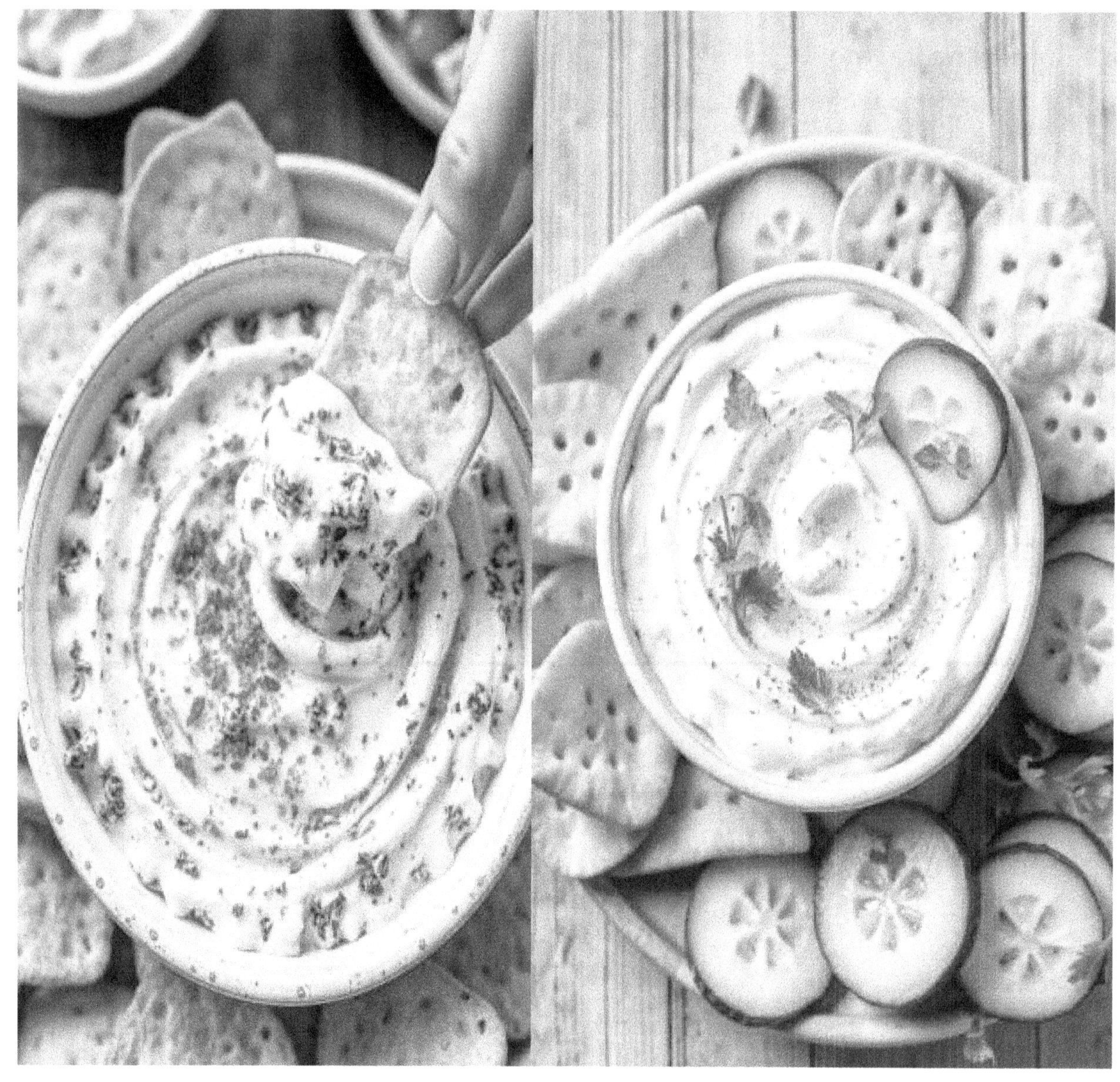

# Hummus and Veggie Platter

Serving: four

Prep Time: 10 minutes

Cooking Time: N/B

## Ingredients:

- For the Hummus:
  - 1 can (15 oz) chickpeas, drained and rinsed
  - 1/4 cup tahini
  - 2 tablespoons olive oil
  - Juice of 1 lemon
  - 2 cloves garlic, minced
  - 1/2 teaspoon ground cumin
  - Salt and black pepper to taste
  - Water, as needed for consistency

## For the Veggie Platter:

  - 1 cucumber, sliced
  - 1 bell pepper, sliced
  - 1 cup cherry tomatoes
  - 1 cup baby carrots
  - 1/2 cup radishes, sliced

## How to Prepare:

1. **Prepare the Hummus:**
   - In a food processor, combine chickpeas, tahini, olive oil, lemon juice, garlic, cumin, salt, and pepper.
   - Process until smooth, adding water a tablespoon at a time until desired consistency is reached.
   - Taste and adjust seasoning as needed.

2. Prepare the Veggies:
   - Arrange sliced cucumber, bell pepper, cherry tomatoes, baby carrots, and radishes on a platter.

3. Serve:
   - Serve hummus in a bowl alongside the veggie platter.

## Ingredients Substitutes and Alternatives:

I. **Tahini:** Use sunflower seed butter or omit for a simpler version.

II. **Chickpeas:** Substitute with white beans or lentils.

## Nutritional Information :

- Calories: 130
- Protein: 5g
- Carbohydrates: 15g
- Dietary Fiber: 4g
- Sugars: 2g
- Fat: 6g
- Saturated Fat: 1g
- Sodium: 200mg
- Potassium: 200mg
- Vitamin C: 10% DV
- Iron: 8% DV

# Baked Sweet Potato Fries

Serving: four

Prep Time: 10 minutes

Cooking Time: 30 minutes

## Ingredients:

- 2 large sweet potatoes, peeled and cut into fries
- 2 tablespoons olive oil
- 1 teaspoon paprika
- 1/2 teaspoon garlic powder
- 1/2 teaspoon onion powder
- 1/2 teaspoon ground cumin
- Salt and black pepper to taste

## How to Prepare:

### 1. Preheat Oven:

❖ Preheat the oven to 425°F (220°C).

### 2. Prepare the Fries:

❖ Toss sweet potato fries with olive oil, paprika, garlic powder, onion powder, cumin, salt, and pepper.

❖ Spread fries in a single layer on a baking sheet.

### 3. Bake the Fries:

❖ Bake for 25-30 minutes, flipping halfway through, or until fries are crispy and golden brown.

### 4. Serve:

❖ Serve hot, with your favorite dipping sauce if desired.

## Ingredients Substitutes and Alternatives:

I. **Sweet Potatoes:** Use regular potatoes or butternut squash.
II. **Spices:** Adjust seasoning to your taste or use a pre-made spice blend.

## Nutritional Information :

- Calories: 180
- Protein: 2g
- Carbohydrates: 30g
- Dietary Fiber: 4g
- Sugars: 7g
- Fat: 6g
- Saturated Fat: 1g
- Sodium: 200mg
- Potassium: 450mg
- Vitamin A: 150% DV
- Vitamin C: 10% DV
- Iron: 6% DV

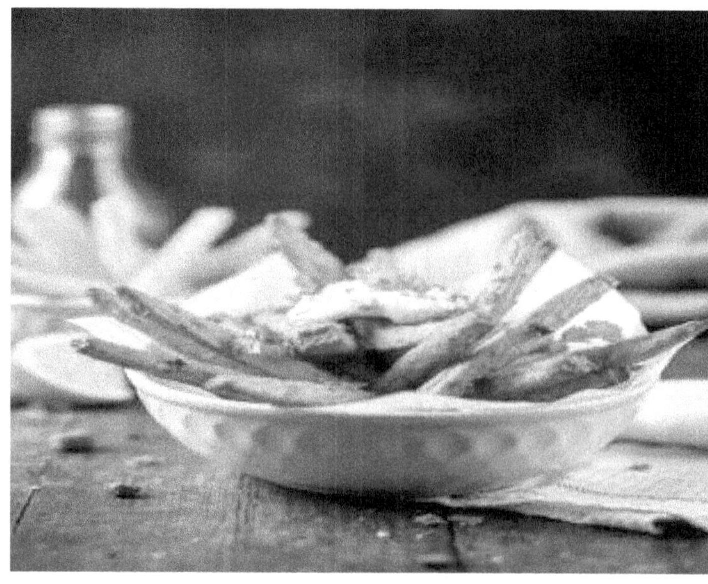

# Spicy Roasted Chickpeas

Serving: 2

Prep Time: 10  minutes

Cooking Time: 15  minutes

## Ingredients:

- 1 can (15 oz) chickpeas, drained and rinsed
- 1 tablespoon olive oil
- 1 teaspoon smoked paprika
- 1/2 teaspoon cayenne pepper (adjust to taste)
- 1/2 teaspoon garlic powder
- 1/2 teaspoon onion powder
- Salt to taste

## How to Prepare:

1. **Preheat Oven:**
   - ❖ Preheat the oven to 400°F (200°C).

2. **Prepare Chickpeas:**
   - ❖ Pat chickpeas dry with a paper towel.
   - ❖ Toss chickpeas with olive oil, smoked paprika, cayenne pepper, garlic powder, onion powder, and salt.

3. **Roast the Chickpeas:**
   - ❖ Spread chickpeas in a single layer on a baking sheet.
   - ❖ Roast for 20-25 minutes, shaking the pan halfway through, until chickpeas are crispy.

4. **Serve:**
   - ❖ Let cool slightly before serving.

## Ingredients Substitutes and Alternatives:

I.   **Chickpeas:** Substitute with other legumes like black beans or lentils.
II.  **Spices:** Adjust spice levels or use a different spice blend.

## Nutritional Information :

- Calories: 120
- Protein: 6g
- Carbohydrates: 18g
- Dietary Fiber: 5g
- Sugars: 2g
- Fat: 3g
- Saturated Fat: 0.5g
- Sodium: 150mg
- Potassium: 250mg
- Vitamin A: 10% DV
- Iron: 10% DV

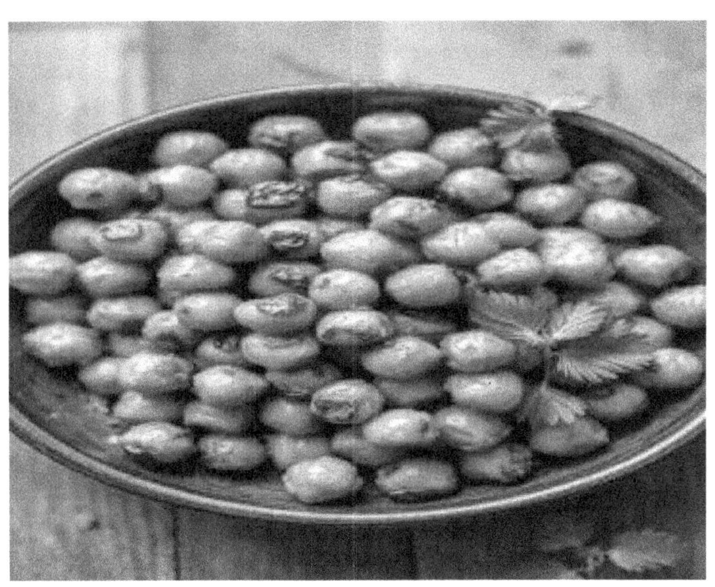

# Caprese Skewers

Serving: four

Prep Time: 10 minutes

Cooking Time: N/B

## Ingredients:

- 1 pint cherry tomatoes
- 8 ounces fresh mozzarella balls (bocconcini)
- Fresh basil leaves
- 2 tablespoons balsamic glaze
- 1 tablespoon olive oil
- Salt and black pepper to taste

## How to Prepare:

1. **Assemble the Skewers:**
   - ❖ On small skewers or toothpicks, thread one cherry tomato, one mozzarella ball, and a basil leaf.

2. **Drizzle and Season:**
   - ❖ Arrange skewers on a serving platter.
   - ❖ Drizzle with balsamic glaze and olive oil.
   - ❖ Season with salt and pepper.

3. **Serve:**
   - ❖ Serve immediately or chill until ready to serve.

## Ingredients Substitutes and Alternatives:

I. **Mozzarella Balls:** Use cubed feta or goat cheese.
II. **Balsamic Glaze:** Substitute with a simple balsamic vinaigrette.

## Nutritional Information:

- Calories: 60
- Protein: 4g
- Carbohydrates: 3g
- Dietary Fiber: 0g
- Sugars: 2g
- Fat: 4g
- Saturated Fat: 2g
- Sodium: 150mg
- Potassium: 150mg
- Vitamin C: 15% DV
- Calcium: 10% DV

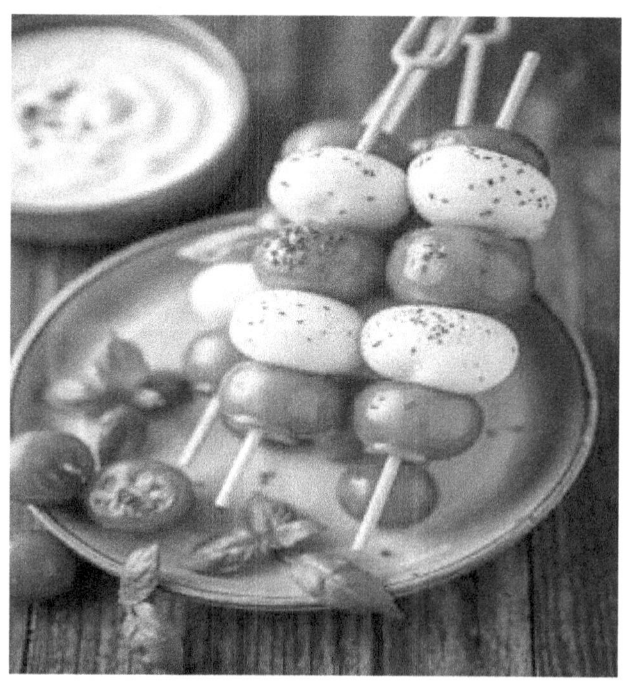

# Avocado and Black Bean Dip

Serving: 2

Prep Time: 10 minutes

Cooking Time: N/B

## Ingredients:

- 1 can (15 oz) black beans, drained and rinsed
- 1 ripe avocado
- 1/4 cup diced red onion
- 1/4 cup chopped cilantro
- Juice of 1 lime
- 1 clove garlic, minced
- Salt and black pepper to taste

## How to Prepare:

1. **Prepare the Dip:**
   - ❖ In a bowl, mash the avocado with a fork.
   - ❖ Stir in black beans, red onion, cilantro, lime juice, garlic, salt, and pepper.

**2. Serve**:
   - ❖ Serve with tortilla chips, pita bread, or fresh vegetables.

## Ingredients Substitutes and Alternatives:

I. **Black Beans:** Use kidney beans or chickpeas.
II. **Avocado:** Substitute with Greek yogurt for a creamier dip.

## Nutritional Information:

- Calories: 130
- Protein: 6g
- Carbohydrates: 18g
- Dietary Fiber: 6g
- Sugars: 1g
- Fat: 6g
- Saturated Fat: 1g
- Sodium: 200mg
- Potassium: 400mg
- Vitamin C: 15% DV
- Iron: 10% DV

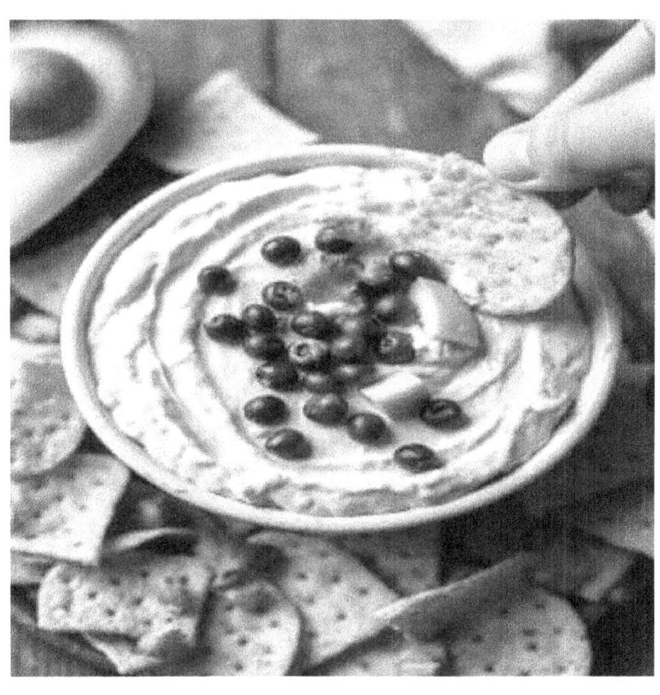

# Greek Yogurt and Cucumber Dip

Serving: 1

Prep Time: 10 minutes

Cooking Time: N/B

## Ingredients:

- 1 cup Greek yogurt (plain, non-fat or low-fat)
- 1/2 cup diced cucumber
- 1 clove garlic, minced
- 1 tablespoon fresh dill, chopped (or 1 teaspoon dried dill)
- 1 tablespoon lemon juice
- Salt and black pepper to taste

## How to Prepare:

### 1. Prepare the Dip:

❖ In a bowl, combine Greek yogurt, cucumber, garlic, dill, lemon juice, salt, and pepper.

### 2. Serve:

❖ Serve with pita bread, crackers, or fresh vegetables.

## Ingredients Substitutes and Alternatives:

I. **Greek Yogurt**: Use regular plain yogurt or a dairy-free alternative.

II. **Dill:** Use parsley or chives.

## Nutritional Information:

- Calories: 50
- Protein: 5g
- Carbohydrates: 5g
- Dietary Fiber: 1g
- Sugars: 3g
- Fat: 2g
- Saturated Fat: 1g
- Sodium: 40mg
- Potassium: 150mg
- Vitamin C: 5% DV
- Calcium: 10% DV

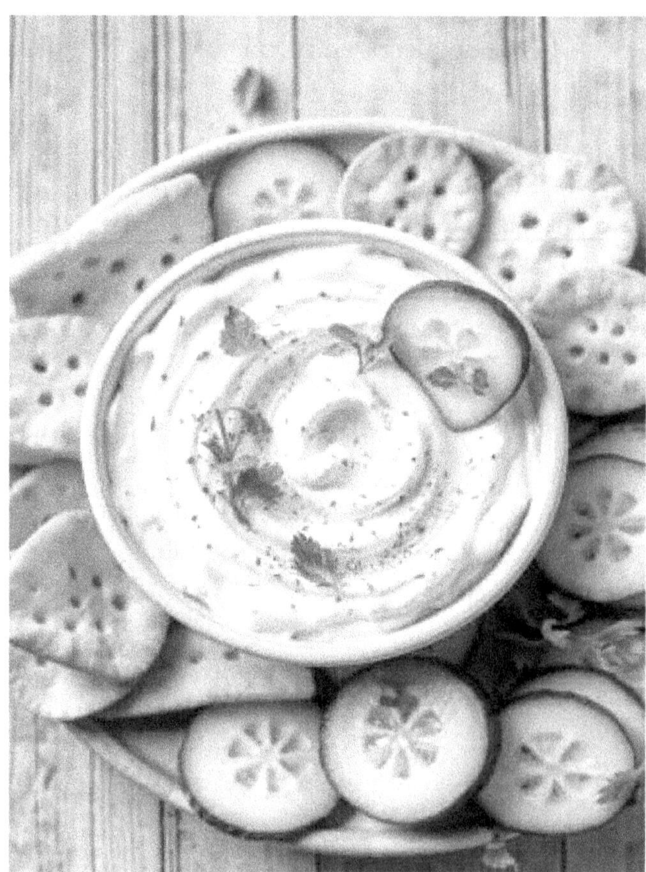

# Roasted Red Pepper Hummus

Serving: 2

Prep Time: 10 minutes

Cooking Time: N/B

## Ingredients:

- 1 can (15 oz) chickpeas, drained and rinsed
- 1/2 cup roasted red peppers (jarred or fresh)
- 1/4 cup tahini
- 2 tablespoons olive oil
- Juice of 1 lemon
- 2 cloves garlic, minced
- 1/2 teaspoon ground cumin
- Salt and black pepper to taste
- Water, as needed for consistency

## How to Prepare:

1. **Prepare the Hummus:**
   - ❖ In a food processor, combine chickpeas, roasted red peppers, tahini, olive oil, lemon juice, garlic, cumin, salt, and pepper.
   - ❖ Process until smooth, adding water as needed to achieve desired consistency.

2. **Serve:**
   - ❖ Serve with pita chips or fresh vegetables.

## Ingredients Substitutes and Alternatives:

I. **Roasted Red Peppers:** Use sun-dried tomatoes or omit for plain hummus.
II. **Tahini:** Use sunflower seed butter or omit.

## Nutritional Information:

- Calories: 130
- Protein: 6g
- Carbohydrates: 18g
- Dietary Fiber: 5g
- Sugars: 3g
- Fat: 6g
- Saturated Fat: 1g
- Sodium: 200mg
- Potassium: 250mg
- Vitamin A: 10% DV
- Iron: 8% DV

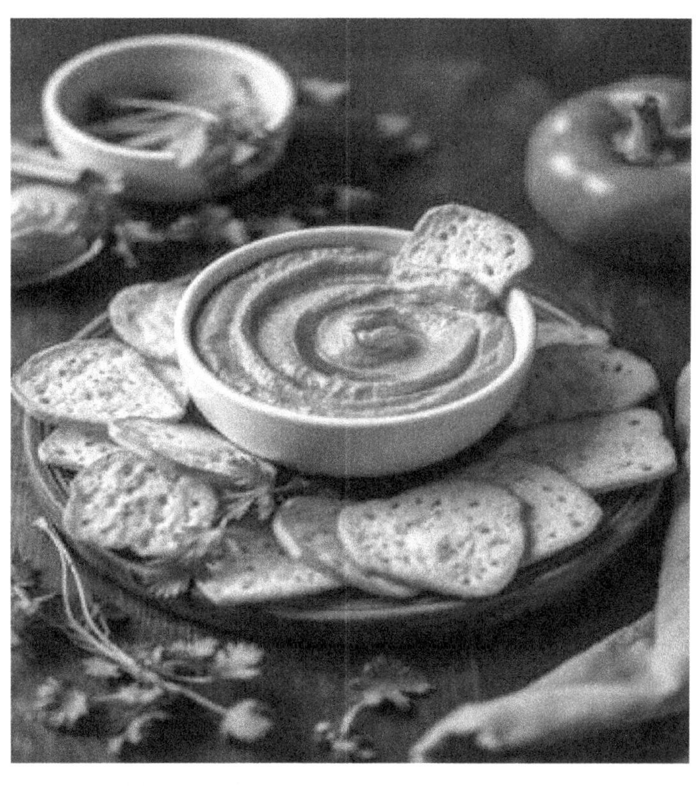

# Stuffed Mini Bell Peppers

Serving: four

Prep Time: 15 minutes

Cooking Time: 20 minutes

## Ingredients:

- 12 mini bell peppers, halved and seeded
- 1 cup cooked quinoa
- 1/2 cup crumbled feta cheese
- 1/4 cup chopped kalamata olives
- 1/4 cup chopped sun-dried tomatoes
- 2 tablespoons chopped fresh basil
- 1 tablespoon olive oil
- Salt and black pepper to taste

## How to Prepare:

1. **Preheat Oven:**
   - ❖ Preheat the oven to 375°F (190°C).

2. **Prepare the Filling:**
   - ❖ In a bowl, combine cooked quinoa, feta cheese, olives, sun-dried tomatoes, basil, olive oil, salt, and pepper.

3. **Stuff the Peppers:**
   - ❖ Spoon filling into each mini bell pepper half.
   - ❖ Arrange stuffed peppers on a baking sheet.

4. **Bake:**
   - ❖ Bake for 15-20 minutes, or until peppers are tender.

5. **Serve:**
   - ❖ Serve warm or at room temperature.

## Ingredients Substitutes and Alternatives:

I. **Quinoa**: Use cooked brown rice or couscous.
II. **Feta Cheese:** Use goat cheese or omit for a dairy-free version.
III. **Kalamata Olives:** Use black olives or green olives.

## Nutritional Information:

- ❖ Calories: 50
- ❖ Protein: 3g
- ❖ Carbohydrates: 6g
- ❖ Dietary Fiber: 1g
- ❖ Sugars: 2g
- ❖ Fat: 2g
- ❖ Saturated Fat: 1g
- ❖ Sodium: 150mg
- ❖ Potassium: 200mg
- ❖ Vitamin A: 30% DV
- ❖ Calcium: 6% DV

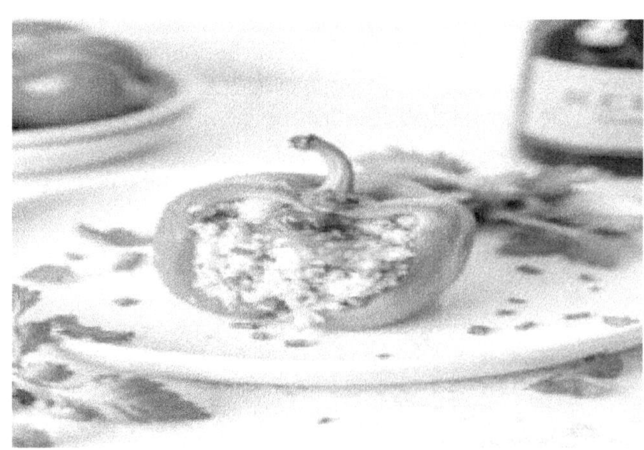

# Spinach and Artichoke Dip

Serving: 2

Prep Time: 10 minutes

Cooking Time: N/B

## Ingredients:

- 1 cup chopped fresh spinach
- 1 cup chopped artichoke hearts (canned or frozen, thawed and drained)
- 1 cup Greek yogurt (plain, non-fat or low-fat)
- 1/2 cup shredded Parmesan cheese
- 1/2 teaspoon garlic powder
- 1/2 teaspoon onion powder
- Salt and black pepper to taste

## How to Prepare:

1. **Prepare the Dip:**
   - ❖ In a bowl, combine spinach, artichoke hearts, Greek yogurt, Parmesan cheese, garlic powder, onion powder, salt, and pepper.
   - ❖ Mix well.

2. **Serve:**
   - ❖ Serve with whole grain crackers, pita bread, or fresh vegetables.

## Ingredients Substitutes and Alternatives:

- ❖ Greek Yogurt: Use sour cream or a dairy-free yogurt.
- ❖ Parmesan Cheese: Use nutritional yeast or omit for a lighter dip.

## Nutritional Information :

- Calories: 80
- Protein: 6g
- Carbohydrates: 6g
- Dietary Fiber: 2g
- Sugars: 3g
- Fat: 4g
- Saturated Fat: 2g
- Sodium: 150mg
- Potassium: 250mg
- Vitamin A: 40% DV
- Calcium: 15% DV

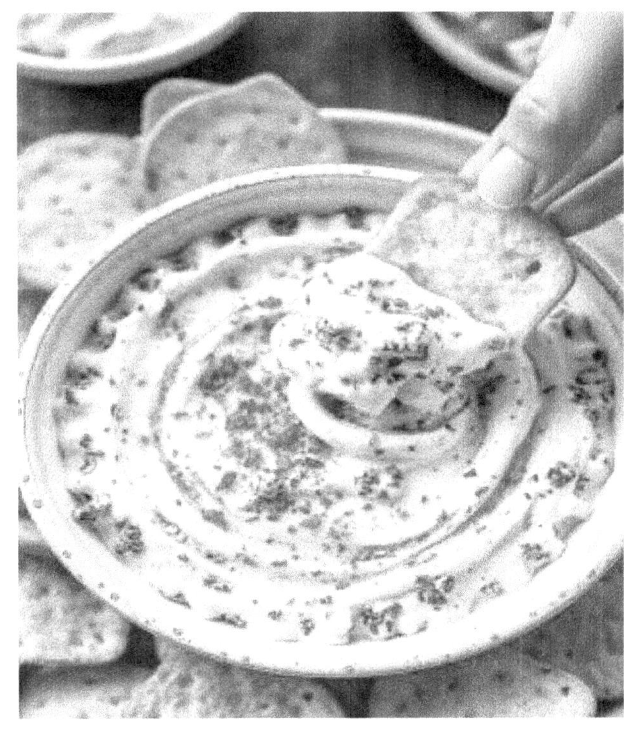

# Baked Zucchini Chips

Serving: four

Prep Time: 10 minutes

Cooking Time: 20 minutes

## Ingredients:

- 2 large zucchinis, sliced thinly
- 1/4 cup whole wheat breadcrumbs
- 1/4 cup grated Parmesan cheese
- 1 teaspoon dried oregano
- 1/2 teaspoon garlic powder
- 1/2 teaspoon onion powder
- 2 tablespoons olive oil
- Salt and black pepper to taste

## How to Prepare:

1. **Preheat Oven:**
   - ❖ Preheat the oven to 425°F (220°C).

2. **Prepare the Zucchini:**
   - ❖ Toss zucchini slices with olive oil, salt, and pepper.
   - ❖ In a separate bowl, mix breadcrumbs, Parmesan cheese, oregano, garlic powder, and onion powder.

3. **Coat and Bake:**
   - ❖ Dip zucchini slices into the breadcrumb mixture and place on a baking sheet in a single layer.
   - ❖ Bake for 15-20 minutes, flipping halfway through, until crispy and golden brown.

4. **Serve:**
   - ❖ Serve hot as a crunchy snack or appetizer.

## Ingredients Substitutes and Alternatives:

I. **Zucchini:** Use yellow squash or eggplant.
II. **Breadcrumbs:** Use gluten-free breadcrumbs or panko.

## Nutritional Information:

- Calories: 100
- Protein: 5g
- Carbohydrates: 10g
- Dietary Fiber: 2g
- Sugars: 4g
- Fat: 5g
- Saturated Fat: 2g
- Sodium: 150mg
- Potassium: 300mg
- Vitamin A: 10% DV
- Calcium: 10% DV

# Chapter 7: Desserts

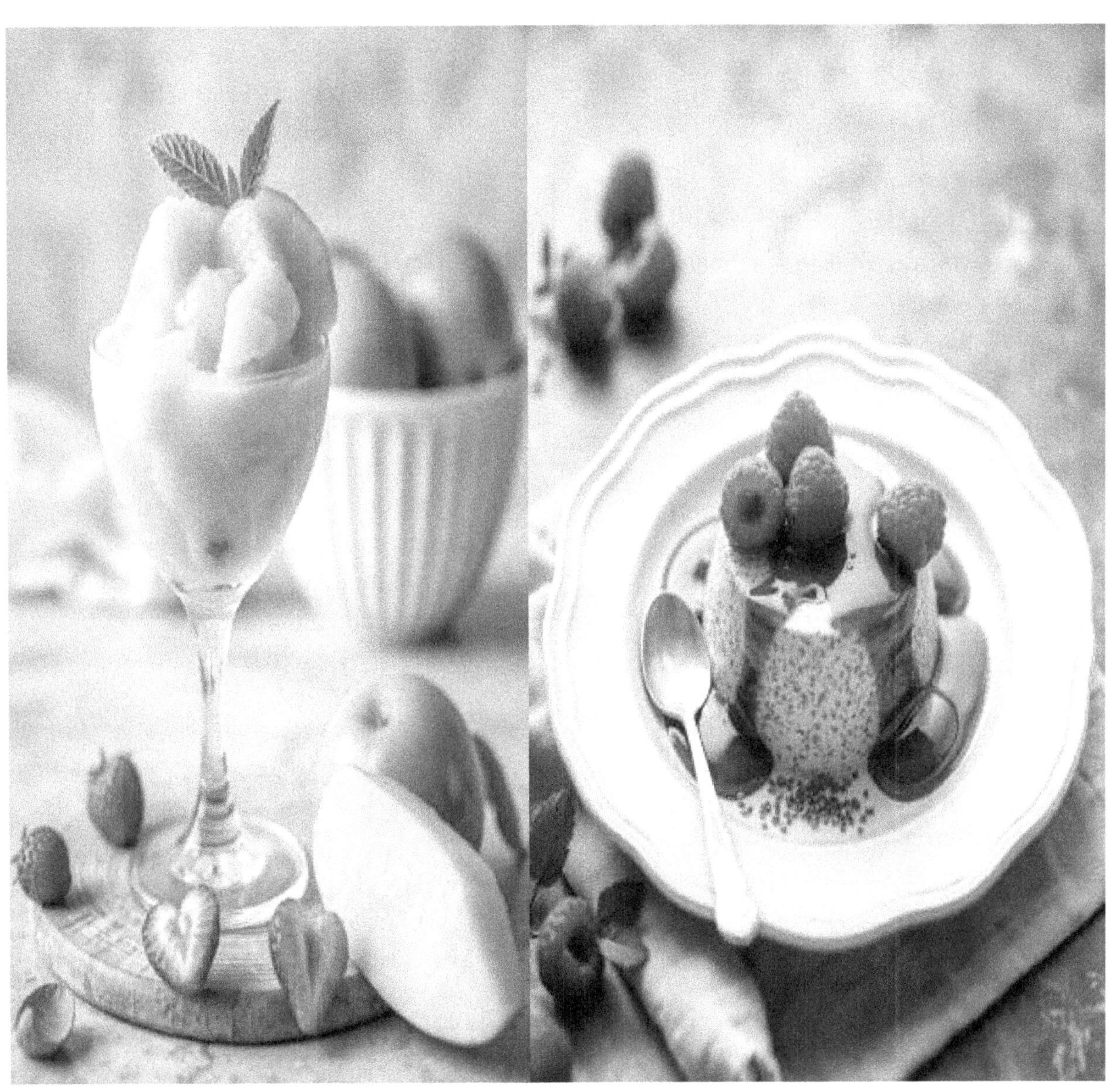

# Fresh Berry Salad

Serving: four

Prep Time: 10 minutes

Cooking Time: N/B

## Ingredients:

- 1 cup strawberries, hulled and halved
- 1 cup blueberries
- 1 cup raspberries
- 1 cup blackberries
- 1 tablespoon honey (or maple syrup)
- 1 tablespoon fresh lemon juice
- Fresh mint leaves for garnish (optional)

## How to Prepare:

### 1. Prepare the Berries:

- ❖ Gently rinse all the berries under cold water and pat dry with paper towels.
- ❖ Combine the strawberries, blueberries, raspberries, and blackberries in a large mixing bowl.

### 2. Make the Dressing:

- ❖ In a small bowl, whisk together honey and lemon juice until well combined.

### 3. Toss and Serve:

- ❖ Drizzle the honey-lemon dressing over the berries and gently toss to coat.
- ❖ Garnish with fresh mint leaves if desired.

## Ingredients Substitutes and Alternatives:

I. **Honey:** Use agave syrup or a sugar substitute.
II. **Berries:** Substitute with any seasonal fruits like peaches, kiwi, or pomegranate seeds.

## Nutritional Information :

- Calories: 80
- Protein: 1g
- Carbohydrates: 20g
- Dietary Fiber: 5g
- Sugars: 15g
- Fat: 0g
- Saturated Fat: 0g
- Sodium: 0mg
- Potassium: 150mg
- Vitamin C: 50% DV
- Iron: 4% DV

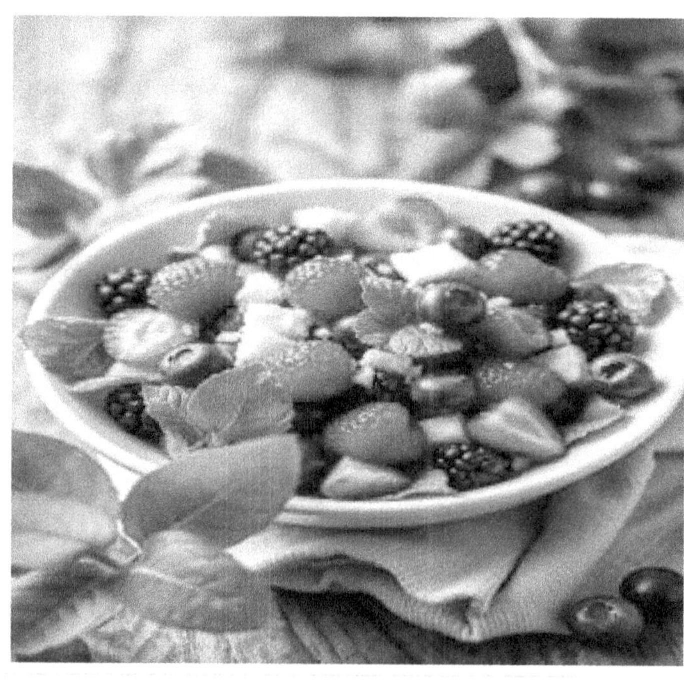

# Dark Chocolate Avocado Mousse

Serving: four

Prep Time: 10 minutes

Cooking Time: N/B

## Ingredients:

- 2 ripe avocados
- 1/4 cup unsweetened cocoa powder
- 1/4 cup pure maple syrup (or honey)
- 1/4 cup almond milk (or any milk of choice)
- 1 teaspoon vanilla extract
- Pinch of salt

## How to Prepare:

1. **Blend the Ingredients:**
   - In a food processor or blender, combine avocados, cocoa powder, maple syrup, almond milk, vanilla extract, and a pinch of salt.
   - Blend until smooth and creamy.

2. **Chill and Serve:**
   - Spoon the mousse into serving dishes and refrigerate for at least 1 hour to firm up.
   - Serve chilled, garnished with fresh berries or a sprinkle of cocoa powder if desired.

## Ingredients Substitutes and Alternatives:

I. **Avocado:** Use silken tofu for a dairy-free alternative.
II. **Maple Syrup:** Use honey or a sugar substitute.

## Nutritional Information:

- Calories: 150
- Protein: 2g
- Carbohydrates: 20g
- Dietary Fiber: 6g
- Sugars: 12g
- Fat: 8g
- Saturated Fat: 1g
- Sodium: 10mg
- Potassium: 400mg
- Vitamin C: 5% DV
- Iron: 8% DV

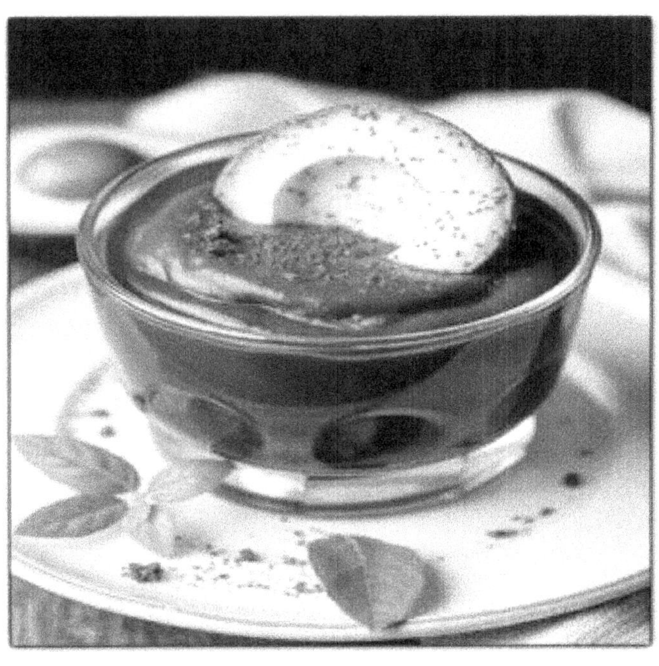

# Baked Apples with Cinnamon

Serving: four

Prep Time: 10 minutes

Cooking Time: 25 minutes

## Ingredients:

- 4 medium apples (such as Honeycrisp or Gala)
- 1/4 cup raisins
- 1/4 cup chopped walnuts (or pecans)
- 2 tablespoons honey
- 1 teaspoon ground cinnamon
- 1/4 teaspoon ground nutmeg

## How to Prepare:

### 1. Preheat Oven:

❖ Preheat the oven to 350°F (175°C).

### 2. Prepare the Apples:

❖ Core the apples, creating a small cavity in the center of each.

❖ In a small bowl, mix raisins, walnuts, honey, cinnamon, and nutmeg.

### 3. Stuff the Apples:

❖ Spoon the mixture into the cavity of each apple.

### 4. Bake:

❖ Place the apples in a baking dish and bake for 20-25 minutes, or until tender.

### 5. Serve:

❖ Serve warm, optionally with a dollop of Greek yogurt or a drizzle of extra honey.

## Ingredients Substitutes and Alternatives:

I. **Apples:** Use pears or peaches.
II. **Raisins:** Substitute with dried cranberries or chopped dates.
III. **Nuts:** Use any preferred nuts or omit.

## Nutritional Information;

- Calories: 180
- Protein: 2g
- Carbohydrates: 35g
- Dietary Fiber: 5g
- Sugars: 25g
- Fat: 5g
- Saturated Fat: 1g
- Sodium: 5mg
- Potassium: 250mg
- Vitamin C: 15% DV
- Iron: 6% DV

# Chia Seed Pudding with Raspberry Sauce

Serving: four

Prep Time: 15 minutes

Cooking Time: 10  minutes

## Ingredients:

For the Chia Seed Pudding:

- 1/4 cup chia seeds
- 1 cup almond milk (or any milk of choice)
- 1 tablespoon maple syrup (or honey)
- 1/2 teaspoon vanilla extract

For the Raspberry Sauce:

- 1 cup fresh or frozen raspberries
- 2 tablespoons honey (or maple syrup)
- 1 tablespoon lemon juice

## How to Prepare:

1. **Prepare the Chia Seed Pudding:**
   - ❖ In a bowl, combine chia seeds, almond milk, maple syrup, and vanilla extract.
   - ❖ Stir well and refrigerate for at least 4 hours or overnight, stirring occasionally until it thickens.

2. **Prepare the Raspberry Sauce**:
   - ❖ In a saucepan, combine raspberries, honey, and lemon juice.
   - ❖ Cook over medium heat, stirring frequently, until raspberries break down and sauce thickens, about 10 minutes.
   - ❖ Let cool.

3. **Assemble and Serve:**
   - ❖ Spoon chia seed pudding into serving dishes and top with raspberry sauce.

## Ingredients Substitutes and Alternatives:

I. **Chia Seeds:** Use flaxseeds for a different texture.
II. **Almond Milk:** Substitute with coconut milk or cow's milk.
III. **Raspberries:** Use strawberries or blueberries.

## Nutritional Information :

- Calories: 160
- Protein: 5g
- Carbohydrates: 22g
- Dietary Fiber: 8g
- Sugars: 10g
- Fat: 7g
- Saturated Fat: 1g
- Sodium: 30mg
- Potassium: 200mg
- Vitamin C: 15% DV
- Calcium: 20% DV

# Almond Flour Brownies

Serving: four

Prep Time: 15 minutes

Cooking Time: 25 minutes

## Ingredients:

- 2 cups almond flour
- 1/2 cup cocoa powder
- 1/2 cup maple syrup (or honey)
- 1/4 cup coconut oil, melted
- 2 large eggs
- 1 teaspoon vanilla extract
- 1/2 teaspoon baking powder
- Pinch of salt

## How to Prepare:

### 1. Preheat Oven:

- ❖ Preheat the oven to 350°F (175°C).

### 2. Prepare the Batter:

- ❖ In a mixing bowl, combine almond flour, cocoa powder, baking powder, and salt.
- ❖ In another bowl, whisk together maple syrup, melted coconut oil, eggs, and vanilla extract.
- ❖ Add wet ingredients to dry ingredients and mix until combined.

### 3. Bake:

- ❖ Pour the batter into a greased 8x8-inch baking pan.
- ❖ Bake for 20-25 minutes, or until a toothpick inserted in the center comes out clean.

### 4. Serve:

- ❖ Let cool before cutting into squares.

## Ingredients Substitutes and Alternatives:

I. **Almond Flour:** Use coconut flour or whole wheat flour.

II. **Maple Syrup:** Use honey or agave syrup.

III. **Coconut Oil:** Substitute with olive oil or butter.

## Nutritional Information:

- Calories: 180
- Protein: 5g
- Carbohydrates: 14g
- Dietary Fiber: 3g
- Sugars: 8g
- Fat: 13g
- Saturated Fat: 6g
- Sodium: 100mg
- Potassium: 150mg
- Vitamin A: 0% DV
- Calcium: 6% DV

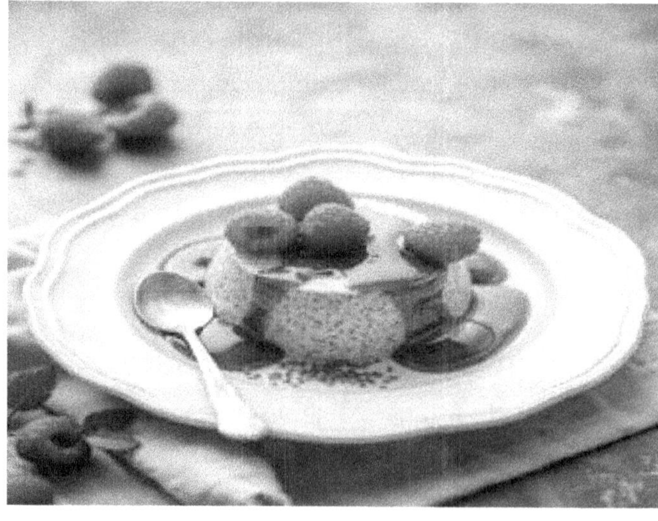

# Lemon Yogurt Cake

Serving: four

Prep Time: 15 minutes

Cooking Time: 35 minutes

## Ingredients:

- 1 cup Greek yogurt (plain, non-fat or low-fat)
- 1/2 cup coconut flour
- 1/2 cup almond flour
- 1/2 cup honey (or maple syrup)
- 3 large eggs
- Zest of 1 lemon
- Juice of 1 lemon
- 1/2 teaspoon baking powder
- Pinch of salt

## How to Prepare:

1. Preheat Oven:
   - Preheat the oven to 350°F (175°C).

2  Prepare the Batter:
   - ❖ In a bowl, whisk together Greek yogurt, honey, eggs, lemon zest, and lemon juice.
   - ❖ In another bowl, mix coconut flour, almond flour, baking powder, and salt.
   - ❖ Combine wet and dry ingredients and mix until smooth.

3. Bake:
   - ❖ Pour batter into a greased 9-inch round cake pan.
   - ❖ Bake for 30-35 minutes, or until a toothpick inserted in the center comes out clean.

4. **Serve:**

   - Let cool before slicing. Optionally, dust with powdered sugar or drizzle with lemon glaze.

## Ingredients Substitutes and Alternatives:

I. **Coconut Flour:** Use all-purpose flour or whole wheat flour.

II. **-Greek Yogurt:** Substitute with regular yogurt or buttermilk.

## Nutritional Information :

- Calories: 150
- Protein: 7g
- Carbohydrates: 18g
- Dietary Fiber: 2g
- Sugars: 12g
- Fat: 7g
- Saturated Fat: 2g
- Sodium: 90mg
- Potassium: 200mg
- Vitamin C: 5% DV
- Calcium: 8% DV

# Banana Oat Cookies

Serving: four

Prep Time: 10 minutes

Cooking Time: 15  minutes

## Ingredients:

- 2 ripe bananas
- 1 cup rolled oats
- 1/2 cup chopped walnuts (or any nuts of choice)
- 1/4 cup dark chocolate chips (optional)
- 1/2 teaspoon vanilla extract
- 1/2 teaspoon ground cinnamon

## How to Prepare:

### 1. Preheat Oven:

❖ Preheat the oven to 350°F (175°C).

### 2. Prepare the Batter:

❖ In a bowl, mash the bananas until smooth.

❖ Stir in oats, walnuts, chocolate chips (if using), vanilla extract, and cinnamon.

### 3. Shape and Bake:

❖ Drop spoonfuls of the mixture onto a baking sheet lined with parchment paper.

❖ Flatten slightly with the back of the spoon.

❖ Bake for 12-15 minutes, or until golden brown.

### 4. Serve:

❖ Let cool on a wire rack before serving.

## Ingredients Substitutes and Alternatives:

I. **Bananas:** Use applesauce or mashed sweet potatoes.

II. **Walnuts:** Use any preferred nuts or omit.

III. **Chocolate Chips:** Substitute with dried fruit or omit.

## Nutritional Information:

- Calories: 80
- Protein: 2g
- Carbohydrates: 12g
- Dietary Fiber: 2g
- Sugars: 6g
- Fat: 3g
- Saturated Fat: 0g
- Sodium: 0mg
- Potassium: 150mg
- Vitamin C: 2% DV
- Calcium: 2% DV

# Mango Sorbet

Serving: four

Prep Time: 10 minutes

freezing Time: 3 hour

## Ingredients:

- 3 cups ripe mango chunks (fresh or frozen)
- 1/2 cup orange juice
- 1/4 cup lime juice
- 1/4 cup honey (or agave syrup)
- Pinch of salt

## How to Prepare:

### 1. Blend Ingredients:

- ❖ In a blender, combine mango chunks, orange juice, lime juice, honey, and salt.
- ❖ Blend until smooth.

### 2. Freeze:

- ❖ Pour the mixture into a shallow dish and freeze for at least 3 hours, stirring occasionally to break up ice crystals.

### 3. Serve:

- ❖ Scoop into bowls and serve.

## Ingredients Substitutes and Alternatives:

I. **Mango**: Use other tropical fruits like pineapple or peaches.

II. **Honey:** Use maple syrup or a sugar substitute.

## Nutritional Information :

- Calories: 100
- Protein: 1g
- Carbohydrates: 26g
- Dietary Fiber: 2g
- Sugars: 22g
- Fat: 0g
- Saturated Fat: 0g
- Sodium: 10mg
- Potassium: 200mg
- Vitamin C: 60% DV
- Calcium: 4% DV

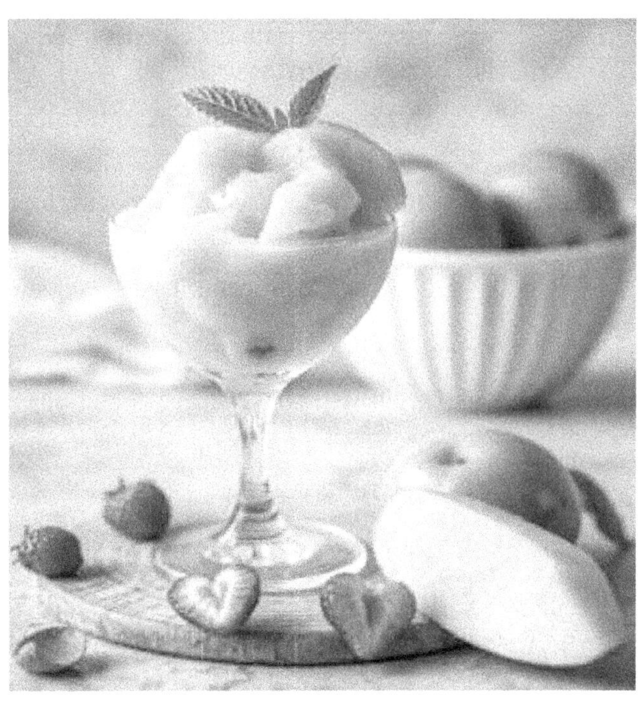

# Carrot Cake Energy Bites

Serving: four

Prep Time: 10 minutes

Cooking Time: N/B

## Ingredients:

- 1 cup rolled oats
- 1/2 cup finely grated carrots
- 1/4 cup raisins
- 1/4 cup chopped walnuts
- 1/4 cup almond butter (or peanut butter)
- 1 tablespoon honey (or maple syrup)
- 1/2 teaspoon ground cinnamon
- 1/4 teaspoon ground ginger
- Pinch of salt

## How to Prepare:

### 1. Mix Ingredients:

❖ In a bowl, combine oats, grated carrots, raisins, walnuts, almond butter, honey, cinnamon, ginger, and salt.

❖ Mix until well combined.

### 2. Form Balls:

❖ Roll the mixture into 1-inch balls and place on a baking sheet lined with parchment paper.

### 3. Chill:

❖ Refrigerate for at least 30 minutes to firm up.

### 4. Serve:

❖ Enjoy as a quick snack or dessert.

## Ingredients Substitutes and Alternatives:

I. Carrots: Use finely grated sweet potatoes or apples.
II. Almond Butter: Use peanut butter or sunflower seed butter.
III. Raisins: Substitute with dried cranberries or chopped dates.

## Nutritional Information:

- Calories: 80
- Protein: 2g
- Carbohydrates: 11g
- Dietary Fiber: 2g
- Sugars: 7g
- Fat: 4g
- Saturated Fat: 1g
- Sodium: 0mg
- Potassium: 150mg
- Vitamin A: 10% DV
- Calcium: 4% DV

# Poached Pears with Vanilla

Serving: four

Prep Time: 10 minutes

Cooking Time: 30  minutes

## Ingredients:

- 4 ripe pears, peeled and cored
- 2 cups water
- 1/2 cup white wine (or apple juice)
- 1/4 cup honey (or agave syrup)
- 1 vanilla bean, split and scraped (or 1 teaspoon vanilla extract)
- 1 cinnamon stick

## How to Prepare:

### 1. Prepare the Poaching Liquid:

- ❖ In a saucepan, combine water, white wine, honey, vanilla bean (or extract), and cinnamon stick.
- ❖ Bring to a simmer over medium heat.

### 2. Poach the Pears:

- ❖ Add the pears to the saucepan and simmer for 15-20 minutes, or until tender.
- ❖ Carefully remove pears and let cool.

### 3. Reduce the Syrup:

- ❖ Continue simmering the poaching liquid until it thickens slightly, about 10 minutes.

### 4. Serve:

- ❖ Drizzle the syrup over the pears before serving.

## Ingredients Substitutes and Alternatives:

I.   **White Wine**: Use apple juice or water.
II.  **Honey:** Substitute with maple syrup or a sugar substitute.

## Nutritional Information:

- Calories: 120
- Protein: 1g
- Carbohydrates: 30g
- Dietary Fiber: 5g
- Sugars: 25g
- Fat: 0g
- Saturated Fat: 0g
- Sodium: 0mg
- Potassium: 200mg
- Vitamin C: 10% DV
- Calcium: 2% DV

# Chapter 8: Special Occasion Meals

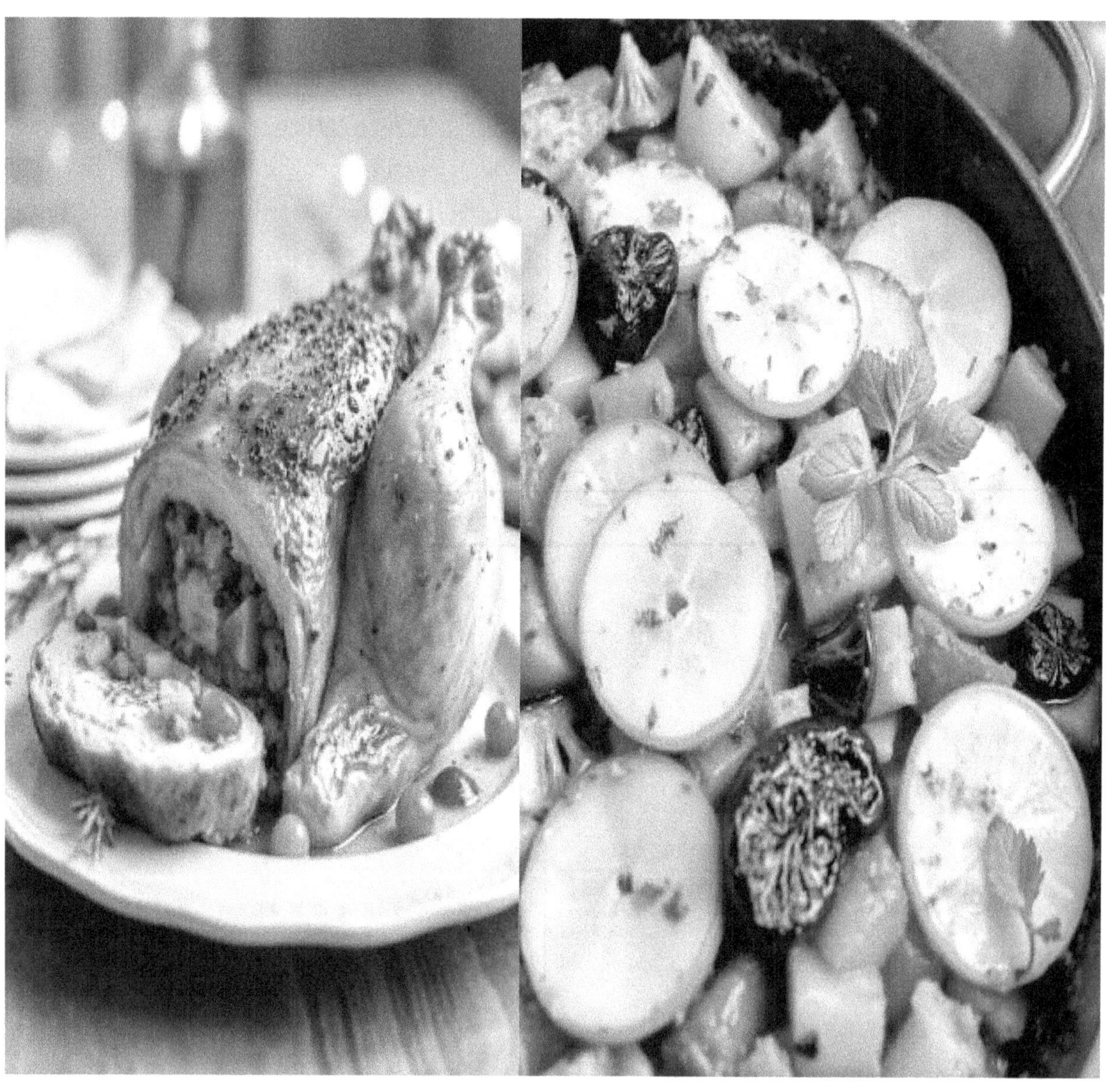

# Herb-Crusted Prime Rib

Serving: 6-8

Prep Time: 15 minutes

Cooking Time: 2 hours and 15 minutes

## Ingredients:

- 1 (4-5 pounds) prime rib roast
- 4 cloves garlic, minced
- 2 tablespoons fresh rosemary, chopped
- 2 tablespoons fresh thyme, chopped
- 2 tablespoons olive oil
- 1 tablespoon Dijon mustard
- 1 tablespoon salt
- 1 teaspoon black pepper
- 1 cup beef broth

## How to Prepare:

1. **Preheat Oven:**
   - ❖ Preheat the oven to 450°F (230°C).

2. **Prepare the Herb Mixture:**
   - ❖ In a small bowl, combine minced garlic, rosemary, thyme, olive oil, Dijon mustard, salt, and black pepper.

3. **Season the Roast:**
   - ❖ Rub the herb mixture evenly over the prime rib roast.

4. **Roast:**
   - ❖ Place the roast in a roasting pan and roast in the preheated oven for 20 minutes.

5. **Reduce Heat:**
   - ❖ Lower the oven temperature to 325°F (165°C) and continue roasting for an additional 1.5-2 hours, or until the internal temperature reaches 130°F (54°C) for medium-rare.

6. **Rest and Serve:**
   - ❖ Remove the roast from the oven and let it rest for 15-20 minutes before carving.
   - ❖ Deglaze the pan with beef broth, scraping up any browned bits to make a delicious gravy.

## Ingredients Substitutes and Alternatives:

I. **Herbs:** Use dried herbs if fresh are unavailable.

II. **Dijon Mustard:** Substitute with whole grain mustard or omit if necessary.

## Nutritional Information :

- Calories: 350
- Protein: 28g
- Carbohydrates: 0g
- Dietary Fiber: 0g
- Sugars: 0g
- Fat: 27g
- Saturated Fat: 10g
- Sodium: 650mg
- Potassium: 550mg
- Vitamin C: 0% DV
- Iron: 15% DV

# Holiday Stuffed Turkey Breast

Serving: 6

Prep Time: 20 minutes

Cooking Time: 50 minutes

## Ingredients:

- 4 pounds turkey breast, boneless and skinless
- 1 cup fresh spinach, chopped
- 1/2 cup dried cranberries
- 1/2 cup walnuts, chopped
- 1/2 cup feta cheese, crumbled
- 1/2 cup breadcrumbs (whole wheat or gluten-free)
- 2 tablespoons olive oil
- 1 teaspoon dried thyme
- 1 teaspoon dried rosemary
- Salt and black pepper, to taste

## How to Prepare:

**1. Prepare the Stuffing:**

- ❖ In a bowl, combine spinach, cranberries, walnuts, feta cheese, breadcrumbs, thyme, rosemary, salt, and pepper.

**2. Prepare the Turkey Breast:**

- ❖ Preheat the oven to 375°F (190°C).
- ❖ Lay the turkey breast flat on a cutting board. Place a piece of plastic wrap over it and gently pound to an even thickness.

**3. Stuff and Roll:**

- ❖ Spread the stuffing mixture evenly over the turkey breast.
- ❖ Roll the turkey breast tightly, securing it with kitchen twine.

**4. Roast:**

- ❖ Heat olive oil in a large ovenproof skillet over medium-high heat.
- ❖ Sear the stuffed turkey breast on all sides until golden brown, about 5 minutes.
- ❖ Transfer the skillet to the preheated oven and roast for 40-50 minutes, or until the internal temperature reaches 165°F (74°C).

**5. Rest and Serve:**

- ❖ Let the turkey rest for 10 minutes before slicing.

## Ingredients Substitutes and Alternatives:

I. **Spinach:** Use kale or Swiss chard.
II. **Cranberries:** Substitute with raisins or dried cherries.
III. **Feta Cheese:** Use goat cheese or omit if dairy-free.

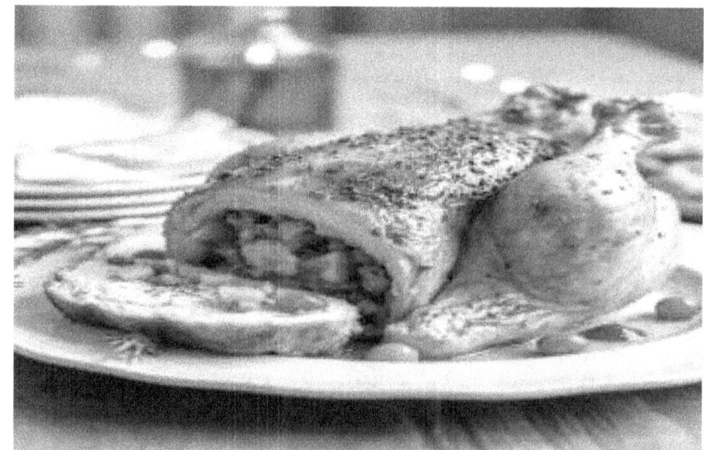

## Nutritional Information:

- Calories: 320
- Protein: 30g
- Carbohydrates: 15g
- Dietary Fiber: 3g
- Sugars: 7g
- Fat: 15g
- Saturated Fat: 4g
- Sodium: 600mg
- Potassium: 450mg
- Vitamin C: 15% DV
- Iron: 10% DV

# Grilled Lobster Tails

Serving: four

Prep Time: 15 minutes

Cooking Time: 10  minutes

## Ingredients:

- 4 lobster tails
- 1/4 cup olive oil
- 2 cloves garlic, minced
- 1 tablespoon lemon juice
- 1 tablespoon fresh parsley, chopped
- Salt and black pepper, to taste

## How to Prepare:

1. **Prepare the Lobster Tails:**
   - ❖ Using kitchen shears, cut the top of the lobster tails lengthwise, from the base to the tip. Carefully lift the meat from the shell, keeping it attached at the base.

2. **Prepare the Marinade:**
   - ❖ In a bowl, mix olive oil, minced garlic, lemon juice, parsley, salt, and pepper.

3. **Marinate the Lobster:**
   - ❖ Brush the lobster meat with the marinade and let it sit for 15 minutes.

4. **Grill:**
   - ❖ Preheat the grill to medium-high heat.
   - ❖ Place lobster tails flesh-side down on the grill and cook for 5-6 minutes.
   - ❖ Flip and cook for an additional 3-4 minutes, or until the meat is opaque and cooked through.

5. **Serve:**
   - ❖ Serve the lobster tails with extra lemon wedges and fresh parsley.

## Ingredients Substitutes and Alternatives:

I. **Olive Oil:** Use melted butter for a richer flavor.
II. **Lemon Juice:** Substitute with lime juice or a splash of white wine.

## Nutritional Information:

- Calories: 220
- Protein: 28g
- Carbohydrates: 1g
- Dietary Fiber: 0g
- Sugars: 0g
- Fat: 11g
- Saturated Fat: 1.5g
- Sodium: 400mg
- Potassium: 300mg
- Vitamin C: 15% DV
- Iron: 10% DV

# Vegetable Paella

Serving: four

Prep Time: 15 minutes

Cooking Time: 30  minutes

## Ingredients:

- 1 tablespoon olive oil
- 1 onion, chopped
- 2 cloves garlic, minced
- 1 red bell pepper, diced
- 1 green bell pepper, diced
- 1 cup green peas (fresh or frozen)
- 1 cup cherry tomatoes, halved
- 1 cup artichoke hearts (canned or frozen), chopped
- 1 1/2 cups short-grain rice
- 3 cups vegetable broth
- 1 teaspoon smoked paprika
- 1/2 teaspoon saffron threads (optional)
- Salt and black pepper, to taste
- Fresh parsley, for garnish

## How to Prepare:

### 1. Prepare the Vegetables:

- ❖ Heat olive oil in a large skillet or paella pan over medium heat.
- ❖ Add onions and garlic, sauté until translucent.

### 2. Add Vegetables:

- ❖ Stir in bell peppers, green peas, cherry tomatoes, and artichoke hearts.
- ❖ Cook for 5-7 minutes until vegetables start to soften.

### 3. Add Rice and Seasonings:

- ❖ Stir in rice, smoked paprika, saffron (if using), salt, and pepper.
- ❖ Pour in vegetable broth and bring to a boil.

### 4. Simmer:

- ❖ Reduce heat to low, cover, and simmer for 20-25 minutes, or until rice is cooked and liquid is absorbed.
- ❖ Remove from heat and let sit for 5 minutes before serving.

### 5. Serve:

- ❖ Garnish with fresh parsley before serving.

<u>**Ingredients Substitutes and Alternatives:**</u>

I. **Vegetable Broth**: Use chicken broth or water.
II. **Rice:** Substitute with quinoa or another short-grain variety.
III. **Artichoke Hearts**: Omit or substitute with olives.

## Nutritional Information :

- Calories: 290
- Protein: 7g
- Carbohydrates: 50g
- Dietary Fiber: 5g
- Sugars: 8g
- Fat: 8g
- Saturated Fat: 1g
- Sodium: 600mg
- Potassium: 600mg
- Vitamin C: 30% DV
- Iron: 15% DV

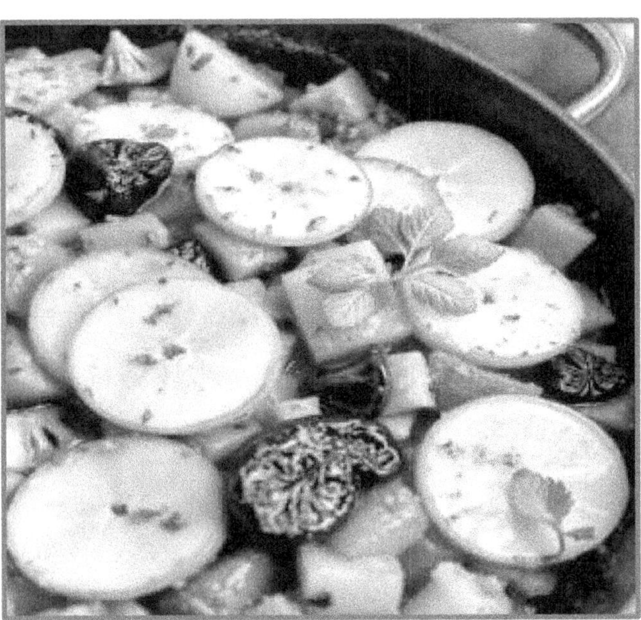

# Spiced Pumpkin Soup

Serving: 6

Prep Time: 10 minutes

Cooking Time: 25 minutes

## Ingredients:

- 1 tablespoon olive oil
- 1 onion, chopped
- 2 cloves garlic, minced
- 1 (15-ounce) can pumpkin puree (or 2 cups fresh pumpkin, roasted and pureed)
- 4 cups vegetable broth
- 1/2 cup coconut milk
- 1 teaspoon ground cumin
- 1/2 teaspoon ground cinnamon
- 1/4 teaspoon ground nutmeg
- Salt and black pepper to taste
- Fresh parsley or chives, for garnish

## How to Prepare:

1. **Prepare the Base**:
   - ❖ Heat olive oil in a large pot over medium heat.
   - ❖ Add onions and garlic, sauté until soft and translucent.

2. **Add Pumpkin and Spices:**
   - ❖ Stir in pumpkin puree, vegetable broth, coconut milk, cumin, cinnamon, nutmeg, salt, and pepper.
   - ❖ Bring to a simmer and cook for 15-20 minutes, stirring occasionally.

3. **Blend the Soup:**

❖ Use an immersion blender to puree the soup until smooth. Alternatively, carefully transfer to a blender in batches.

4. **Serve:**

❖ Garnish with fresh parsley or chives before serving.

## Ingredients Substitutes and Alternatives:

I. **Pumpkin Puree**: Use butternut squash or sweet potato puree.

II. **Coconut Milk:** Substitute with regular milk or a dairy-free alternative.

## Nutritional Information :

- Calories: 150
- Protein: 3g
- Carbohydrates: 22g
- Dietary Fiber: 5g
- Sugars: 6g
- Fat: 6g
- Saturated Fat: 5g
- Sodium: 600mg
- Potassium: 500mg
- Vitamin A: 80% DV
- Calcium: 6% DV

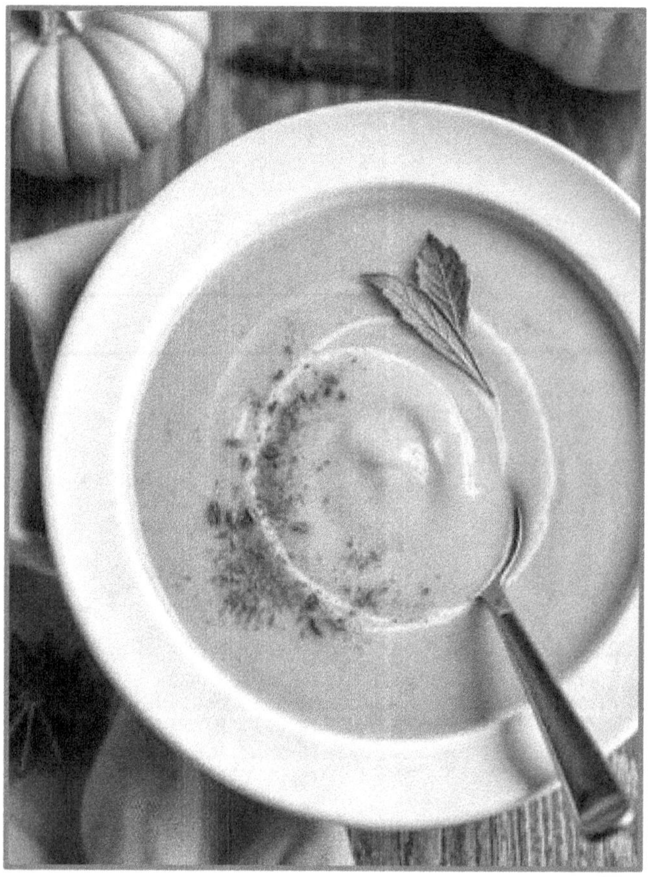

# 60 Days Meal Plan

**Day 1:**

- Breakfast: Avocado Toast with Poached Egg
- Lunch: Quinoa and Black Bean Salad
- Dinner: Baked Salmon with Dill
- Snack: Almond Flour Brownies
- Beverage: Herbal Iced Tea

**Day 2:**

- Breakfast: Blueberry Oatmeal with Almonds
- Lunch: Mediterranean Chickpea Bowl
- Dinner: Beef and Barley Stew
- Snack: Caprese Skewers
- Beverage: Citrus Infused Water

**Day 3:**

- Breakfast: Fresh Fruit and Yogurt Parfait
- Lunch: Roasted Beet and Orange Salad
- Dinner: Grilled Lemon Herb Chicken
- Snack: Chia Seed Pudding with Mango
- Beverage: Classic Tomato Juice

**Day 4:**

- Breakfast: Banana Oat Cookies
- Lunch: Greek Salad with Feta
- Dinner: Moroccan Lamb Tagine
- Snack: Hummus and Veggie Platter
- Beverage: Strawberry Basil Lemonade

**Day 5:**

- Breakfast: Apple Cinnamon Quinoa
- Lunch: Warm Lentil and Sweet Potato Salad
- Dinner: Grilled Shrimp Skewers
- Snack: Roasted Red Pepper Hummus
- Beverage: Warm Turmeric Golden Milk

**Day 6:**

- Breakfast: Whole Wheat Pancakes with Berries
- Lunch: Spicy Chickpea and Avocado Salad
- Dinner: Stuffed Bell Peppers
- Snack: Fresh Berry Salad
- Beverage: Refreshing Cucumber Mint Water

**Day 7:**

- Breakfast: Almond Butter and Banana Smoothie
- Lunch: Kale and Apple Salad with Walnuts
- Dinner: Mushroom and Barley Soup

- Snack: Baked Zucchini Chips

- Beverage: Herbal Iced Tea

**Day 8:**

- Breakfast: Spinach and Feta Omelette

- Lunch: Chicken Tortilla Soup

- Dinner: Quinoa Stuffed Acorn Squash

- Snack: Carrot Cake Energy Bites

- Beverage: Classic Tomato Juice

**Day 9:**

- Breakfast: Chia Seed Pudding with Raspberry Sauce

- Lunch: Roasted Brussels Sprouts with Balsamic Glaze

- Dinner: Turkey and Spinach Meatballs

- Snack: Baked Sweet Potato Fries

- Beverage: Citrus Infused Water

**Day 10:**

- Breakfast: Smoked Salmon and Cream Cheese Bagel

- Lunch: Minestrone Soup

- Dinner: Spicy Tofu Stir-Fry

- Snack: Dark Chocolate Avocado Mousse

- Beverage: Strawberry Basil Lemonade

**Day 11:**

- Breakfast: Greek Yogurt with Honey and Walnuts

- Lunch: Garlic and Herb Mashed Cauliflower

- Dinner: Herb-Crusted Prime Rib

- Snack: Roasted Red Pepper Hummus

- Beverage: Warm Turmeric Golden Milk

**Day 12:**

- Breakfast: Tropical Paradise Smoothie

- Lunch: Butternut Squash Soup

- Dinner: Grilled Lobster Tails

- Snack: Poached Pears with Vanilla

- Beverage: Refreshing Cucumber Mint Water

**Day 13:**

- Breakfast: Fresh Fruit and Yogurt Parfait

- Lunch: Spicy Black Bean Soup

- Dinner: Holiday Stuffed Turkey Breast

- Snack: Almond Flour Brownies

- Beverage: Herbal Iced Tea

**Day 14:**

- Breakfast: Apple Cinnamon Quinoa

- Lunch: Classic Caesar Salad with a DASH Twist

- Dinner: Baked Salmon with Dill

- Snack: Hummus and Veggie Platter

- Beverage: Classic Tomato Juice

**Day 15:**

- Breakfast: Blueberry Oatmeal with Almonds

- Lunch: Lentil and Spinach Stew

- Dinner: Stuffed Mini Bell Peppers

- Snack: Fresh Berry Salad

- Beverage: Citrus Infused Water

**Day 16:**

- Breakfast: Whole Wheat Pancakes with Berries

- Lunch: Warm Lentil and Sweet Potato Salad

- Dinner: Beef and Barley Stew

- Snack: Dark Chocolate Avocado Mousse

- Beverage: Strawberry Basil Lemonade

**Day 17:**

- Breakfast: Banana Oat Cookies

- Lunch: Kale and Apple Salad with Walnuts

- Dinner: Moroccan Lamb Tagine

- Snack: Roasted Zucchini Chips

- Beverage: Herbal Iced Tea

**Day 18:**

- Breakfast: Almond Butter and Banana Smoothie

- Lunch: Mediterranean Chickpea Bowl

- Dinner: Grilled Lemon Herb Chicken

- Snack: Chia Seed Pudding with Mango

- Beverage: Warm Turmeric Golden Milk

**Day 19:**

- Breakfast: Spinach and Feta Omelette

- Lunch: Garlic and Herb Mashed Cauliflower

- Dinner: Spicy Tofu Stir-Fry

- Snack: Carrot Cake Energy Bites

- Beverage: Refreshing Cucumber Mint Water

**Day 20:**

- Breakfast: Smoked Salmon and Cream Cheese Bagel

- Lunch: Mushroom and Barley Soup

- Dinner: Quinoa Stuffed Acorn Squash

- Snack: Poached Pears with Vanilla

- Beverage: Classic Tomato Juice

**Day 21:**

- Breakfast: Chia Seed Pudding with Raspberry Sauce

- Lunch: Roasted Brussels Sprouts with Balsamic Glaze

- Dinner: Grilled Shrimp Skewers

- Snack: Fresh Berry Salad

- Beverage: Citrus Infused Water

**Day 22:**

- Breakfast: Fresh Fruit and Yogurt Parfait

- Lunch: Spicy Chickpea and Avocado Salad

- Dinner: Herb-Crusted Prime Rib

- Snack: Almond Flour Brownies

- Beverage: Strawberry Basil Lemonade

**Day 23:**

- Breakfast: Greek Yogurt with Honey and Walnuts

- Lunch: Butternut Squash Soup

- Dinner: Holiday Stuffed Turkey Breast

- Snack: Baked Sweet Potato Fries

- Beverage: Warm Turmeric Golden Milk

**Day 24:**

- Breakfast: Apple Cinnamon Quinoa

- Lunch: Classic Caesar Salad with a DASH Twist

- Dinner: Baked Salmon with Dill

- Snack: Roasted Red Pepper Hummus

- Beverage: Refreshing Cucumber Mint Water

**Day 25:**

- Breakfast: Tropical Paradise Smoothie

- Lunch: Spicy Black Bean Soup

- Dinner: Grilled Lobster Tails

- Snack: Dark Chocolate Avocado Mousse

- Beverage: Herbal Iced Tea

**Day 26:**

- Breakfast: Whole Wheat Pancakes with Berries

- Lunch: Mediterranean Chickpea Bowl

- Dinner: Chicken Tortilla Soup

- Snack: Poached Pears with Vanilla

- Beverage: Classic Tomato Juice

**Day 27:**

- Breakfast: Chia Seed Pudding with Mango

- Lunch: Garlic and Herb Mashed Cauliflower

- Dinner: Moroccan Lamb Tagine

- Snack: Caprese Skewers

- Beverage: Citrus Infused Water

**Day 28:**

- Breakfast: Blueberry Oatmeal with Almonds

- Lunch: Quinoa and Black Bean Salad

- Dinner: Beef and Barley Stew

- Snack: Fresh Berry Salad

- Beverage: Strawberry Basil Lemonade

**Day 29:**

- Breakfast: Fresh Fruit and Yogurt Parfait

- Lunch: Spicy Chickpea and Avocado Salad

- Dinner: Stuffed Bell Peppers

- Snack: Dark Chocolate Avocado Mousse

- Beverage: Warm Turmeric Golden Milk

**Day 30:**

- Breakfast: Almond Butter and Banana Smoothie

- Lunch: Roasted Beet and Orange Salad

- Dinner: Grilled Lemon Herb Chicken

- Snack: Carrot Cake Energy Bites

- Beverage: Refreshing Cucumber Mint Water

**Day 31:**

- Breakfast: Spinach and Feta Omelette

- Lunch: Warm Lentil and Sweet Potato Salad

- Dinner: Spicy Tofu Stir-Fry

- Snack: Baked Zucchini Chips

- Beverage: Classic Tomato Juice

**Day 32:**

- Breakfast: Greek Yogurt with Honey and Walnuts

- Lunch: Roasted Brussels Sprouts with Balsamic Glaze

- Dinner: Grilled Shrimp Skewers

- Snack: Poached Pears with Vanilla

- Beverage: Citrus Infused Water

**Day 33:**

- Breakfast: Tropical Paradise Smoothie

- Lunch: Kale and Apple Salad with Walnuts

- Dinner: Herb-Crusted Prime Rib

- Snack: Almond Flour Brownies

- Beverage: Strawberry Basil Lemonade

**Day 34:**

- Breakfast: Chia Seed Pudding with Raspberry Sauce

- Lunch: Greek Salad with Feta

- Dinner: Holiday Stuffed Turkey Breast

- Snack: Fresh Berry Salad

- Beverage: Warm Turmeric Golden Milk

**Day 35:**

- Breakfast: Whole Wheat Pancakes with Berries

- Lunch: Minestrone Soup

- Dinner: Chicken Tortilla Soup

- Snack: Caprese Skewers

- Beverage: Refreshing Cucumber Mint Water

**Day 36:**

- Breakfast: Blueberry Oatmeal with Almonds

- Lunch: Quinoa Stuffed Acorn Squash

- Dinner: Moroccan Lamb Tagine

- Snack: Carrot Cake Energy Bites

- Beverage: Classic Tomato Juice

**Day 37:**

- Breakfast: Fresh Fruit and Yogurt Parfait

- Lunch: Warm Lentil and Sweet Potato Salad

- Dinner: Spicy Black Bean Soup

- Snack: Dark Chocolate Avocado Mousse

- Beverage: Citrus Infused Water

**Day 38:**

- Breakfast: Apple Cinnamon Quinoa

- Lunch: Roasted Beet and Orange Salad

- Dinner: Grilled Lemon Herb Chicken

- Snack: Baked Sweet Potato Fries

- Beverage: Herbal Iced Tea

**Day 39:**

- Breakfast: Smoked Salmon and Cream Cheese Bagel

- Lunch: Spicy Chickpea and Avocado Salad

- Dinner: Grilled Lobster Tails

- Snack: Fresh Berry Salad

- Beverage: Strawberry Basil Lemonade

**Day 40:**

- Breakfast: Greek Yogurt with Honey and Walnuts

- Lunch: Garlic and Herb Mashed Cauliflower

- Dinner: Herb-Crusted Prime Rib

- Snack: Roasted Red Pepper Hummus

- Beverage: Warm Turmeric Golden Milk

**Day 41:**

- Breakfast: Tropical Paradise Smoothie

- Lunch: Butternut Squash Soup

- Dinner: Holiday Stuffed Turkey Breast

- Snack: Caprese Skewers

- Beverage: Refreshing Cucumber Mint Water

**Day 42:**

- Breakfast: Almond Butter and Banana Smoothie

- Lunch: Kale and Apple Salad with Walnuts

- Dinner: Spicy Tofu Stir-Fry

- Snack: Poached Pears with Vanilla

- Beverage: Classic Tomato Juice

**Day 43:**

- Breakfast: Chia Seed Pudding with Mango

- Lunch: Quinoa and Black Bean Salad

- Dinner: Spicy Black Bean Soup

- Snack: Fresh Berry Salad

- Beverage: Citrus Infused Water

**Day 44:**

- Breakfast: Whole Wheat Pancakes with Berries

- Lunch: Greek Salad with Feta

- Dinner: Baked Salmon with Dill

- Snack: Roasted Red Pepper Hummus

- Beverage: Warm Turmeric Golden Milk

**Day 45:**

- Breakfast: Fresh Fruit and Yogurt Parfait
- Lunch: Spicy Chickpea and Avocado Salad
- Dinner: Beef and Barley Stew
- Snack: Dark Chocolate Avocado Mousse
- Beverage: Strawberry Basil Lemonade

**Day 46:**

- Breakfast: Spinach and Feta Omelette
- Lunch: Garlic and Herb Mashed Cauliflower
- Dinner: Grilled Shrimp Skewers
- Snack: Carrot Cake Energy Bites
- Beverage: Refreshing Cucumber Mint Water

**Day 47:**

- Breakfast: Banana Oat Cookies
- Lunch: Mediterranean Chickpea Bowl
- Dinner: Quinoa Stuffed Acorn Squash
- Snack: Baked Zucchini Chips
- Beverage: Classic Tomato Juice

**Day 48:**

- Breakfast: Blueberry Oatmeal with Almonds
- Lunch: Classic Caesar Salad with a DASH Twist
- Dinner: Grilled Lemon Herb Chicken

- Snack: Chia Seed Pudding with Raspberry Sauce
- Beverage: Citrus Infused Water

**Day 49:**

- Breakfast: Almond Butter and Banana Smoothie
- Lunch: Spicy Black Bean Soup
- Dinner: Stuffed Bell Peppers
- Snack: Fresh Berry Salad
- Beverage: Strawberry Basil Lemonade

**Day 50:**

- Breakfast: Smoked Salmon and Cream Cheese Bagel
- Lunch: Warm Lentil and Sweet Potato Salad
- Dinner: Moroccan Lamb Tagine
- Snack: Almond Flour Brownies
- Beverage: Warm Turmeric Golden Milk

**Day 51:**

- Breakfast: Chia Seed Pudding with Mango
- Lunch: Roasted Beet and Orange Salad
- Dinner: Herb-Crusted Prime Rib
- Snack: Hummus and Veggie Platter
- Beverage: Refreshing Cucumber Mint Water

**Day 52:**

- Breakfast: Tropical Paradise Smoothie

- Lunch: Minestrone Soup

- Dinner: Holiday Stuffed Turkey Breast

- Snack: Poached Pears with Vanilla

- Beverage: Classic Tomato Juice

**Day 53:**

- Breakfast: Fresh Fruit and Yogurt Parfait

- Lunch: Spicy Chickpea and Avocado Salad

- Dinner: Beef and Barley Stew

- Snack: Caprese Skewers

- Beverage: Citrus Infused Water

**Day 54:**

- Breakfast: Greek Yogurt with Honey and Walnuts

- Lunch: Warm Lentil and Sweet Potato Salad

- Dinner: Baked Salmon with Dill

- Snack: Dark Chocolate Avocado Mousse

- Beverage: Strawberry Basil Lemonade

**Day 55:**

- Breakfast: Spinach and Feta Omelette

- Lunch: Garlic and Herb Mashed Cauliflower

- Dinner: Grilled Shrimp Skewers

- Snack: Fresh Berry Salad

- Beverage: Warm Turmeric Golden Milk

**Day 56:**

- Breakfast: Apple Cinnamon Quinoa

- Lunch: Classic Caesar Salad with a DASH Twist

- Dinner: Spicy Tofu Stir-Fry

- Snack: Baked Zucchini Chips

- Beverage: Refreshing Cucumber Mint Water

**Day 57:**

- Breakfast: Chia Seed Pudding with Raspberry Sauce

- Lunch: Quinoa and Black Bean Salad

- Dinner: Spicy Black Bean Soup

- Snack: Carrot Cake Energy Bites

- Beverage: Classic Tomato Juice

**Day 58:**

- Breakfast: Whole Wheat Pancakes with Berries

- Lunch: Roasted Brussels Sprouts with Balsamic Glaze

- Dinner: Moroccan Lamb Tagine

- Snack: Hummus and Veggie Platter

- Beverage: Citrus Infused Water

**Day 59:**

- Breakfast: Smoked Salmon and Cream Cheese Bagel

- Lunch: Kale and Apple Salad with Walnuts

- Dinner: Beef and Barley Stew

- Snack: Almond Flour Brownies

- Beverage: Herbal Iced Tea

**Day 60:**

- Breakfast: Greek Yogurt with Honey and Walnuts

- Lunch: Spicy Chickpea and Avocado Salad

- Dinner: Grilled Lobster Tails

- Snack: Fresh Berry Salad

- Beverage: Warm Turmeric Golden Milk

# CONCLUSION

## Maintaining a DASH Diet Lifestyle

A significant step toward enhancing your general health and well-being is to follow the DASH diet. The DASH diet, in contrast to many restrictive diets, emphasizes diversity, balance, and nutrient-rich meals that are not only good for your heart but also tasty. As we get to the end of our DASH diet adventure, it's important to think about how you may continue this lifestyle and fully benefit from it in the long run.

## Useful Advice for Sticking to the DASH Diet

Adhering to a DASH diet regimen requires more than just doing as instructed; it also entails making long-lasting adjustments that blend into your regular activities. The following useful advice will assist you in staying on course:

1. **Make a plan ahead:** Organizing your meals is essential to following the DASH diet consistently. Every week, set aside time to make a grocery list, plan your meals, and prepare some ingredients ahead of time. Having wholesome options close at hand lessens the incentive to choose less nourishing options.

2. **Emphasize Variety:** Take advantage of the diversity of foods available to you as part of the DASH diet. Change up your veggies, give new whole grains a try, and play around with different herbs and spices. This guarantees that you're getting a wide variety of nutrients and also makes your meals interesting.

3. **Control Your Sodium Levels**; Lowering salt intake is essential to the DASH diet. Watch out for hidden sodium in restaurant meals, sauces, and processed foods. You have more control over how much sodium you eat when you cook more often at home. When dining out, don't be afraid to request that your food be made with less salt.

4. **Maintain Hydration:** In addition to being beneficial for general health, drinking enough water helps lower blood pressure. Ensure that you consume eight glasses of water or more each day. As tasty substitutes for sugar-filled drinks, try herbal teas or water flavored with fruits and herbs.

5. **Make Mindful Food Choices**: You can enjoy food more and avoid overeating by being mindful of what you eat and how you feel while eating. Enjoy each bite, take your time, and pay attention to your body's hunger and fullness cues.

6. **Include Physical Exercise:** While nutrition plays a big role in health, frequent exercise is just as vital. Aim for 150 minutes or more per week of moderate-to-intense exercise.

Select a regular activity that you enjoy doing, such as yoga, walking, cycling, or swimming, and include it in your daily routine.

7. **Ask for Help:** Support from friends, family, or a community organization can go a long way toward helping one stick to the DASH diet. Talk to others about your objectives, and trade recipes, and support one another in sticking to your schedule.

# Accepting the Long-Term Obligation

The DASH diet is a lifestyle shift that calls for dedication and consistency rather than a quick remedy. But the benefits of persevering make the work worthwhile. Your overall quality of life, mental clarity, and energy levels should all improve with time. There's a chance that your tastes will change as well, becoming more appreciative of healthy foods' inherent flavors.

Remind yourself that it's normal to occasionally stray from the diet. You must stick to the DASH diet's tenets and keep your health as your priority. Results are long-lasting when little, regular improvements are made.

In summary, one of the best methods to promote heart health, control weight, and lower your risk of chronic diseases is to follow a DASH diet lifestyle. You're investing in a better future for yourself and your loved ones by incorporating this diet into your everyday routine. Savor the trip, accept the advantages, and keep learning about the mouthwatering opportunities the DASH diet presents.

# AUTHOR'S REQUEST

Dear Reader,

Thank you for choosing "**The Complete DASH Diet Cookbook for Beginners**" as a guide on your journey to better health. I sincerely hope that the recipes, tips, and insights in this book have inspired you to adopt the DASH diet and make lasting, positive changes in your life.

Your feedback is incredibly valuable to me. If you've enjoyed the book or found it helpful, I would greatly appreciate it if you could take a moment to leave an honest review. Your thoughts not only help me improve future editions but also assist other readers in discovering the benefits of the DASH diet.

Thank you for your support, and I wish you continued success on your path to better health!!